Governing University Hospitals in a Changing Environment

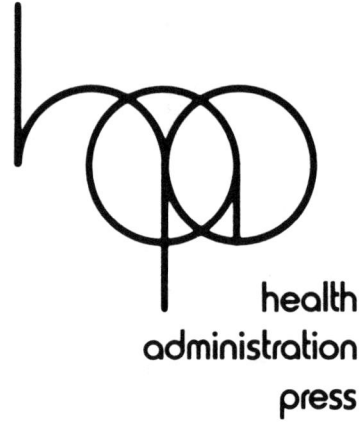

health
administration
press

Editorial Board

John R. Griffith
The University of Michigan

Gordon D. Brown
University of Missouri-Columbia

R. Hopkins Holmberg
Boston University

Arnold D. Kaluzny
University of North Carolina

Carl Meilicke
University of Alberta

Stephen M. Shortell
Northwestern University

David G. Warren
Duke University

Health Administration Press was established in 1972 with the support of the W.K. Kellogg Foundation and is a nonprofit endeavor of The University of Michigan Program and Bureau of Hospital Administration.

THOMAS CHOI
ROBERT F. ALLISON
FRED MUNSON

Governing University Hospitals in a Changing Environment

Health Administration Press
Ann Arbor, Michigan
1986

Copyright © 1986 by the Regents of The University of Michigan. Printed in the United States of America. All rights reserved. This book or parts thereof may not be reproduced in any form without written permission of the publisher.

Library of Congress Cataloging in Publication Data

Choi, Thomas.
    Governing university hospitals in a changing environment.

    Includes index.
    1. Hospitals, University—Administration. 2. Hospitals, Teaching—Administration. I. Allison, Robert F. II. Munson, Fred C. III. Title. [DNLM: 1. Hospitals, Teaching—organization & administration—United States. 2. Social Change—United States. 3. Social Conditions—United States.
WX 27 AA1C5g]
RA975.U5C48   1986   362.1'1'068   85-17688
ISBN   0-910701-10-5

Health Administration Press
School of Public Health
The University of Michigan
1021 East Huron
Ann Arbor, Michigan 48109
(313) 764-1380

In appreciation of our mothers.

Contents

	Foreword	ix
	Preface	xiii
Chapter 1	Introduction and Synopsis	1
Chapter 2	Issues, Theory, and Methodology	9
Chapter 3	University Hospitals and Their Environment	27
Chapter 4	Measuring University Hospital Performance	53
Chapter 5	Structure of the Political Environment	67
Chapter 6	Testing the Limits of the State Environment	85
Chapter 7	The Impact of the Environment on University Hospital Performance: An Explanatory Model	99

Chapter 8	The Financial Viability of University-Owned Hospitals	117
Chapter 9	Managing Support Services in University Hospitals	137
Chapter 10	Medical Staff Organization and Patient Care	151
Chapter 11	Governance and Management of University Hospitals	173
Chapter 12	Conclusions	191
Appendix A	Survey Questionnaire	207
Appendix B	Survey and Field Study Respondents	217
	Index	221

Foreword

Few institutions in our society are as poorly understood as the hospital. The riddle of the hospital, to paraphrase Churchill, is further wrapped in mystery when it comes to our knowledge of the workings of the teaching hospital. This all-important institution, the site of medical education, the venue of the most complex attention for the sickest patients, and the home of vastly disproportionate amounts of care for the poor, is fundamental to the advance and progress of medicine. Like other hospitals, the teaching institution is faced with radical changes in its environment, especially its funding. As payers move to systems in which they pay the same price for care regardless of the type of hospital in which it is delivered, the teaching hospital becomes more and more vulnerable and its future less and less secure. Given this background, this book is of special consequence. It presents a rigorous examination, based on substantial empirical evidence, of the operations and governance of the teaching hospital.

Choi, Allison, and Munson report here their findings from a study of the 52 university-owned teaching hospitals that cooperated in this effort through a special consortium of university hospitals formed to advance this work. The book focuses on the issues of governance and management. As such it touches the two most important areas of deficiency in existing hospital literature. By using sophisticated statistical methods, the authors truly advance our understanding of the basic relationships among trustees, professional administrators, state legislatures, and physicians in their interactions and attempts at controlling the future of the hospital. It is in these relationships that the hospital derives its strength as an institution. In light of this, the authors wisely have examined the personal motivations of the various actors. By combining what are essentially anthropological and sociological methods with motivational analysis, they have produced a first class institutional analysis that any student of hospitals would do well to consider.

Indeed, this book may be as important for its methods as it is for its subject. Despite its importance in American society, consuming roughly 5 percent of gross national product, our conceptual understanding of the hospital as an institution and its importance to society is minimal. This may strike the reader as impossible, given the number of university programs in hospital administration, virtually all of which are run on the graduate level. However, for years the curriculum of these programs has focused on the "how to" of running hospitals, with no emphasis on developing a theoretical understanding of the institution itself. The research product of faculty in these programs has been directed, for the most part, at questions that would make the administration of hospitals more efficient—improved personnel strategies, increased efficiency in food services, reducing accounts receivable, and so on. The presence of graduate programs in business is a strong analog to hospital administration in this respect. Research literature centers on managerial problem solving rather than on a theoretical understanding of business itself. Much of this negligence has been excused on the misguided notion that academic economics was concerning itself with such pursuits. In fact, economics threw off institutional studies so long ago in favor of macroeconomic model building that institutional analysis is viewed as illegitimate in most economics departments. That is why it is important to have Choi, Allison, and Munson, all of whom are connected with university programs in health research, produce a thoroughgoing institutional analysis, using quantitative methods, which offers substantial new wisdom on hospital behavior.

In their approach they have relied heavily on the path-breaking work of the late James D. Thompson who added greatly to our conceptual understanding of the behavior of complex organizations like hospitals. His notion that the work of management was to prepare for the future of the organization and that in complex institutions it is critical to find meaningful measures of progress lest the organization lull itself into a sense of preparedness when in fact it is doomed to extinction is enormously apt to the task of this book. The reader will do well to appreciate that conceptualization of Thompson is advanced by the authors in their efforts to really get inside the teaching hospital.

The immediate future for teaching hospitals in general is uncertain at best. Other hospitals, gradually investing in the technology that was once the hallmark of the teaching hospital, speak frankly about taking "market share" away from these institutions. Because of their location in inner cities where they have been part of a symbiosis with the poor, the pursuit of an ambiguous service/teaching/survival identity, and the absence of large financial reserves, the typical teaching hospital appears ill-equipped to make or even meet its future. Recognizing the difference in input factor costs and the particular expenses of their teaching missions, the federal government currently provides a significant Medicare differential to teaching institutions. This differential will be the subject of enormous concern in the future. The Commonwealth Foundation, in an effort to advance understanding around the problem of ensuring the future of the nation's teaching hospitals as special preserves for training, research, and complex tertiary care, has invested in a major research program designed, among other things, to examine the true costs of graduate medical education supported by the hospital. As government budgets tighten and as employers, unions, and insurance companies design new programs aimed at reducing hospital costs, the teaching hospital will have a difficult time persuading payers, and ultimately society, that the function it serves is worth substantially more than what patients and insurors pay for care in other hospitals.

The work in hand takes us well down the road to understanding the organization of the teaching hospital and what the institution must do to ensure its future. The great test of the contribution of this book will be whether the parties, when equipped with new knowledge, will behave any differently. Personally, I am hopeful. The authors have added significantly to our knowledge of the internal dynamics of the hospital as decisions are made. This information should be used to facilitate organizational change. Equally important, however, is the challenge they present to scholars who follow to turn their attention to institutional behavior as a legitimate subject of hospital analysis.

CARL J. SCHRAMM, PH.D., J.D.

Associate Professor of
Health Policy and Management
Johns Hopkins University
School of Hygiene and Public Health

Director
Johns Hopkins Center for
Hospital Finance and Management

Preface

Since a university hospital is so complex, each one has justifiably argued its uniqueness. Until very recently this sense of uniqueness has gone unchallenged because these hospitals did not meet as a common forum. However, the combination of market pressures and increasing governance and management complexities demanded that university hospitals assess their common problems and goals. So in January 1980 a small group of university hospital administrators and researchers met to discuss these issues. The organization of the meeting was spearheaded by John W. Westerman, then Executive Director of the University of Minnesota Hospitals and Clinics, with help from two other prominent university hospital directors: Jeptha W. Dalston of University of Michigan Hospitals, and Roy S. Rambeck, then of the University of Washington Hospitals, currently retired.

The meeting served two major purposes: for hospital administrators to form a consortium through which to present challenging issues of hospital governance and management, and for researchers to respond with a research protocol. As a result, The Consortium for the Study of University Hospitals (CSUH) was founded; it funded the research which began in 1981. The research intent was twofold: to report to CSUH the study findings and to make visible those issues affecting university hospitals by means of scholarly publications.

Researchers invited to the January 1980 meeting were from different institutions: Gerald E. Bisbee from the American Hospital Association, Thomas Choi and John E. Kralewski from the University of Minnesota, Fred Munson from the University of Michigan, Robin S. MacStravic and Stephen M. Shortell from the University of Washington. Members from the three universities were asked to conduct the project. After Scott MacStravic and Stephen Shortell left the University of Washington, Robert F. Allison from Wayne State University was invited to join the research team. Professor Allison was a logical choice as he was knowledgeable about university hospital governance and management, and has had first-hand experience with it. The research team was then made up of Bob Allison, Fred Munson, and myself, with Fred Munson as project director.

Robert Allison had much earlier recognized the important influence of the state's political culture and economic wealth on its state-owned university hospitals. He was tireless in his effort to find data measuring this influence. His insight on the nature of state influence also helped refine the definition of a state-owned university hospital's ownership environment. The state's role became a focal point throughout our book; his insights were independently verified by Carl Schramm's article on state support and teaching hospitals, which appeared in a 1983 volume of the *New England Journal of Medicine.* Allison presented and elaborated on the notion of state influence in chapters 3 and 5, for which he assumed primary responsibility. He made further good use of our interview data and took primary responsibility for chapter 10 as well.

John R.C. Wheeler and Bridget C. Booske helped our efforts greatly by contributing chapter 8 on university hospital finance. They were able to adopt our theoretical framework and made appropriate use of our data.

Three other chapters were written with help from Stephen Hinkamp (chapter 4), William Kerr (author of the section on strategies in chapter 9), Mark Mantei and Diane Bischak (chapter 11), and John Ives (chapter 2). John Ives, Executive Vice-President of William A. Shands Teaching Hospital and Clinics (University of Florida at Gainesville), succeeded John Westerman as President of CSUH when the study was conducted. His contribution to chapter 2 was only a small portion of his efforts devoted to making the job of the researchers easier.

We wish to acknowledge the many university hospitals that responded to our survey and especially to the 15 university hospitals that opened their doors to us to conduct extensive interviews in preparation for the survey. (A reproduction of the survey and the list of university hospitals that responded are to be found in appendix A.) Some of the respondents are members of CSUH, others are not. Without their cooperation, this study would not have been possible. Similarly, we thank those who permitted us to collect secondary data, including administrators in individual hospitals and the Council of Teaching Hospitals of the Association of American Medical Colleges (AAMC), state census bureaus, and the American Hospital Association. We particularly wish to note the gracious cooperation of Richard M. Knapp and Joseph C. Isaacs in releasing data to us from AAMC, once such data were permitted for release from each hospital.

Laura Pitt at the Center for Health Services Research, University of Minnesota, handled the massive data from these diverse sources, and worked with remarkable skill and forbearance to meet the researchers' incessant requests for computer outputs against impending deadlines.

We wish also to thank our study steering committee, which was composed of:

Donald B. Clapp, J.D.
Vice-President for Administration
University of Kentucky

William B. Deal, M.D.
Dean
College of Medicine
University of Florida at Gainesville

John Ives
President, CSUH
Executive Vice-President
William A. Shands Teaching Hospital and Clinics
University of Florida at Gainesville

William N. Kelley, M.D.
Chairman
Department of Internal Medicine
School of Medicine
University of Michigan

Paul G. Quie, M.D.
Chief of Staff
University of Minnesota Hospitals and Clinics

Neal A. Vanselow, M.D.
Then Chancellor and Vice-President
College of Medicine
University of Nebraska
Currently Vice-President for Health Sciences
University of Minnesota

The members of the steering committee deserve special thanks. They were patient when we needed time to acquaint ourselves with the issues, and pointed us in the proper direction when we asked for advice. They helped us interpret our observations and gave their time freely. In short, it was an excellent steering committee, both critical and supportive.

We wish to thank Jane Telleen, whose editorial assistance enlivened our prose and introduced order and uniformity to our manuscript. We also want to thank our wives, Elaine Allison, Leslie Gillette, and Mary Munson. During the many occasions when we descended upon each other's homes, they tempered the intensity of our work with grace, despite pressing projects of their own. Finally, we wish to thank CSUH formally for its funding, and to thank the Bush Foundation for additional support.

T.C.
Minneapolis

ONE

Introduction and Synopsis

INTRODUCTION

This introduction contains a brief essay on the issues confronting university hospitals, followed by a synopsis of each chapter in the book.

Essay: The Issues

In addition to the provision of care to patients, university hospitals establish a setting for clinical research and medical education. While these three missions help shape the character of university hospitals, what defines the uniqueness of university hospitals is their ownership. University hospitals, both privately and publicly owned, operate under the overall regulations and expectations of academia. Public or state-owned university hospitals, and to a lesser extent privately owned university hospitals, are subject also to the interests and expectations of the state in which they are located. States, universities, and faculty all have vested interests in these institutions and may make owner-like claims on the hospitals (e.g., care for indigents, advancing research, teaching, and innovative health care). Therefore, decisions that affect the hospital are not the exclusive domain of those who manage it, but are shared with—if not subjugated to—the different owner groups.

The nature and type of decisions to be made, by whom, and at what level are issues of governance that traditionally did not require much attention until competition from the commercial sector increased. Furthermore, when new federal and state policies encouraged health care competition, those people closely associated with university hospitals became concerned that support for their institutions may be eroding. There are those who would argue that university hospitals are ill-equipped to compete against the commercial sector because of the teaching and research costs added to patient care. Others would argue that the traditional governance of the host university and its hospital should be made separate. Simultaneous governance of both the university and hospital by the same policy-making group (e.g., university regents) is quite acceptable as long as there is sufficient financial support for the hospital. That is, a hospital in a financially supportive environment renders the form of governance relatively unimportant. But if university hospitals are expected to fend for themselves by being competitive or efficient, they would need the attention of a streamlined governing body that is knowledgeable about health care issues, whose express attention is centered on the complexities of health care competition, and that is authorized to make policy decisions for these hospitals quickly—or at least in pace with the fast-changing conditions of a competitive climate.

Satisfying the owners is one thing, and being able to compete with other providers is another. If what owners want and what hospital survival requires are at odds, university hospitals will be forced to make adaptive changes. The nature of these changes lodges in the ability of university hospitals to adapt to competitive demands quickly and to anticipate them. The traditional form of university hospital governance has therefore been subjected to scrutiny. The elaborate decision-making process endemic to academic institutions does not meet the needs of hospitals caught in a turbulent environment. The following example may serve to illustrate a point: a chief executive officer in a large, private, multihospital chain—who earlier served in the same capacity in a university hospital—was asked what was the most striking difference between the two jobs. His response: "Decisions now seem too easy. Each time I walk out of a decision-making session, I always feel that there must be some key group I neglected to get approval from."

If federal and state support for educational and research functions is very limited, this will in effect force university hospitals to become more commercial. Some university hospital physicians may then find it more appropriate to work in the commercial sector. Such a migration will further compound the competitive pressure on the university hospital as tertiary care physicians leave to aid competitors. A timely illustration of many of the large issues confronting university hospitals is the fact that Dr. William C. DeVries, who performed the first artificial heart transplant on Dr. Barney Clark, left the University of Utah to become a part of Humana Inc., a for-profit organization. Whether Dr. DeVries left because he grew tired of waiting for another approval from the university to perform a second heart implantation, as the media alleged, is secondary to the fact that he did leave, like many physicians before him and no doubt many to come.

Facing a change in hospital governance is only one step in the direction of making the university hospital a more independent entity. There are those who are concerned that this may set the university hospital in a drift away from academia. Concerns about too much independence, or even incipient commercialization, are not trivial. The dilemma many university hospitals currently face is either to emulate the commercial sector or accept mounting financial pressures. The emulation of the commercial corporate world is not without consequence. It will probably make university hospitals better equipped to compete, but perhaps at the expense of their educational and research emphases. In some ways the university hospitals face a winless situation. Without commercialization, they find themselves increasingly unable to adapt to a competitive environment. With commercialization, however, their character will probably change. In either event, as financial pressures mount and support services and equipment ebb, physicians associated with university hospitals find it less difficult to join the competitive commercial sector.

A change in traditional governance may be seen as an adaptive response of the university hospital. Interestingly enough, those university hospitals that enjoy changing forms of governance already are doing relatively well financially. And where necessary their state officials will help keep them solvent. These states traditionally have supported health, education, and welfare proactively—that is, with initiative. Conversely, hospitals in less proactive states either have to instigate support from the ownership environment, or forcibly try to cut themselves loose in order to thrive as a corporation independent from the university and its system of governance.

In short, university hospitals are increasingly bound by their environments. To the extent that their environments—that is, ownership and competition—are inconsistent, they will need to adapt. The adaptive functions fall squarely on the nature of governance and the corporate structure of the hospital.

The above provides a backdrop for this study. It is based on carefully designed theory-based research and corresponding rigorous meth-

4 / *Governing University Hospitals*

ods of analysis that safeguard against random injection of subjective bias and also enable others to test and replicate our findings in other settings.

For these reasons, we have taken pains in these chapters to describe in detail how we framed our study theoretically, and how we collected and analyzed our data. For those who simply wish to bypass the details of the study, an overall sense of our findings is provided in the synopsis below.

SYNOPSIS

This book reports on a study of university hospitals in the United States that has policy implications for the governance and management of these hospitals.

Data for the study were collected from multiple sources: (1) published statistical data from the American Hospital Association for 1980, Association of American Medical Colleges (AAMC), the Census Bureau, and various states; (2) financial and operating data authorized by individual university hospitals and provided for 1979–81 by the Council of Teaching Hospitals, AAMC; (3) intensive field studies of 15 university hospitals stratified by various factors such as geographical location and hospital size. Interviewees in this study included university regents, presidents, chief executive officers of hospitals, state legislators, clinical chiefs of staff, university administrative officials, hospital advisory board members, allied health personnel, and competitors; (4) primary data gathered in 1982 from questionnaire responses by 52 of the 64 public and private university-owned hospitals in the United States.

Issues, Theory, and Methodology

Chapter 2 clarifies the characteristics of university hospitals, and spells out the issues confronting them, the organizational theories that help explain their circumstances, and the methods used to study them. This chapter describes how the shifting health care environment has decreased the university hospital's dominance in the tertiary care market—making it but one of several major competitors. The current change in the health care environment demands a concomitant change in the governance and management functions of the university hospital, so that it may become more adaptive to prevailing environmental constraints.

Three theories of organizations, each giving a special perspective, may be used to explain the challenge of governing and managing university hospitals. The first perspective sees university hospitals as dependent on resources from the environment. The increasing competition for scarce resources forces many nonuniversity hospitals to react by reorganizing or by corporate restructuring (e.g., the formation of multihospital systems). The university hospital, however, being structurally embedded in the larger network of the university and the state, is not in a position to make similar adjustments.

The second perspective sees university hospitals as having achieved a certain level of organizational inertia—a consequence of their previous achievements and dominance. This inertia renders the university hospital unable to adapt to the fast-changing environment. According to this theory, organizations reach the end of their organizational life cycle because they are unable to deviate from the fixed routines that initially brought them prominence.

The third perspective challenges such a deterministic perspective, defining university hospitals as protected institutions by virtue of their history, tradition, and embodiment of state values and pride. Thus, the state provides protective insulation that alleviates the market pressures rendering university hospitals vulnerable under the first and second models. That is, pure market conditions may constrain but not necessarily devastate a state-supported institution.

Finally, chapter 2 briefly outlines the several methods used for data analyses, foremost among which are the causal modeling techniques of path analysis and factor analysis. As subsequent chapters show, the causal models explain how university hospitals situated in highly proactive states (characterized by an active legislature, strong emphasis on health, education, and welfare, and support for them) are most protected and least likely to founder because of financial exigencies.

University Hospitals and Their Environment

Chapter 3 describes several types of environment: the market environment, the political environment, the ownership environment, and the environment internal to the university hospital. The external environments are shown to affect the governance and management structures and functions of the university hospital. Included in this discussion are the size and composition of governing boards, board proactivity, decision-making groups, and the shifting loci of decision-making power.

Measuring University Hospital Performance

Chapter 4 deals with complications related to the measurement of hospital performance, our dependent variable. Performance is of two types: efficiency and hospital viability. The efficiency index is a measure of how efficiently facilities, operating capital, and materials are used. Viability is defined in two ways: the amount of net revenues (including state appropriations) over total operating expenses; a second definition excludes appropriations from the numerator. The fact that these two measures are used does not imply that there is a set of universally agreed-upon measures for performance. Reasons accounting for the complexities of measuring performance are elaborated.

Structure of the Political Environment

Chapter 5 deals in depth with the multiple indicators used to measure the state's political environment. These indicators are factored into a highly reliable scale. The chapter starts with a historical perspective on the relationship between the university hospital and the state, and then classifies the political environment into three different subcultures: moralist, elitist, and individualist. The chapter then shows the empirical relationships between the political environment and several variables critical to university hospital viability. Policy implications are drawn for hospital governance in various political and market environments.

Testing the Limits of the State Environment

Chapter 6 deals with an extended systematic test of the impact of both the political and market environment on the viability of the university hospital, the length of chief executive officer (CEO) tenure, and the comprehensiveness of state support for charity care. Results indicate that university hospitals in more proactive states are better protected. But protection in any state, provided by the owners, sometimes comes with a price: that of ownership constraints. The university hospital has to satisfy many parties, some of which are quite diverse, if not conflicting. Such constraints are shown to have some effect on shortening the tenure of university hospital chief executive officers.

The Impact of the Environment on University Hospital Performance: An Explanatory Model

Chapter 7 presents a causal model of successive effects emanating from the state environment that eventually influence hospital performance. The model explains 46 percent of the variations in hospital viability and 37 percent of the variations in hospital efficiency. It is significant that while the state environment clearly affects the medical school, a high-ranking medical school, with its teaching obligations, has no significant deleterious effect on hospital efficiency (beta or path coefficient

= −0.085) and in fact helps university hospital viability (0.174). Similarly, a proactive state that pays for welfare significantly helps the viability of university hospitals (0.296). However, a state that pays for welfare also tends to create disincentive for efficiency (−0.131). Competition, in contrast, tends to create incentive for greater efficiency (0.293) but insignificantly affects viability (−0.060). A governing board that takes initiatives tends to encourage management to pay attention to the environment (0.265), which in turn positively affects efficiency (0.305) and viability (0.153).

Discussions of the results cover many facets, but the foremost is that university hospitals in proactive states are protected institutions, not likely to be devastated by the forces and consequences of unbridled competition. From a policy standpoint, these institutions can best maximize their viability by keeping a positive, healthy relationship with the state.

The Financial Viability of University-Owned Hospitals

Chapter 8 presents additional causal models showing the impact of different variables such as hospital size, efficiency, number of admissions, capital financing, indigent care, case mix, and type of payment source on hospital costs and financial viability. One model explains 77 percent of the variations in hospital costs. Significant factors contributing to costs are hospital size, admissions, efficiency, input prices, and the degree of indigent care. The financial viability of university hospitals is closely related to the level of gross revenues, costs, and collection rates. The level of state support is particularly important to state-owned university hospitals.

Also noteworthy is the difference between privately and publicly owned university hospitals. Privately owned university hospitals showed higher levels of occupancy during 1981 but they also had higher levels of debt, largely because they did not receive as much state financial support—thus necessitating greater use of the debt market for raising capital.

Managing Support Services in University Hospitals

Chapter 9 presents the first of several chapters devoted to the application of data and findings in actual management situations. The chapter explains why the hospital administration's reputation often depends on the successful management of support services, and why the management of such services in the university hospital setting is particularly difficult.

Medical Staff Organization and Patient Care

Chapter 10 analyzes the relationship between the medical school (structure and faculty) and patient care provided in the university hospital under different types of political and market conditions. Factors that affect patient care include: the faculty's medical service plan, the governance of the medical school faculty, the patient care decision-making process, and the nature of institutional leadership.

Governance and Management of University Hospitals

Chapter 11 discusses managerial and governance tensions and conflicts—namely, between the hospital and its university—and suggests some solutions. This discussion provides five major observations: (1) state support is important but state control often accompanies such support; state control is less pronounced in proactive states; (2) university influence on university hospitals is strong and has several specific advantages; (3) there is perpetual tension between the university's desire to control the hospital for educational purposes and the hospital's desire for greater autonomy in order to meet an increasingly competitive environment. This tension accounts for a significant part of the hospital governance problem; (4) a possible solution to these problems is to give the hospital autonomy by channeling all significant influence (from state government, the university administration, the medical school, and the community) through a strong hospital-specific governing board, and to give control to the university through its control of membership on that board; (5) if this solution is implemented, it will likely strengthen the role of hospital administration but weaken the influence of other groups.

Conclusions

Chapter 12 closes the book with an overall retrospective and prospective analysis of the centrality of the ownership environment, the changing character of competition, the prospective payment system, the role of hospital governance, and the composition and effectiveness of governing boards.

TWO

Issues, Theory, and Methodology

At least since the late 1970s, directors of state university hospitals have been coping with an environment more harsh and turbulent than they could have predicted. Many of them have been particularly worried that their management and governance structures are ill-equipped to meet the challenges posed by the changing health care environment they face every day. Even worse, perhaps, is their fear that things are changing so fast they will not be able to adjust quickly enough under the traditional form of university hospital governance.

Indeed, their fears are not unfounded. Consider the implications for university hospitals of the following changes in health care:

- Specialized services such as corneal and heart transplants, once found almost exclusively at university hospitals, are now being provided by more specialists in the community.
- Medical schools and other health-education programs can now look to other facilities if the university hospital cannot accommodate their students or their teaching needs.
- With the increase of external controls (such as state regulations and competition from other health care organizations), university hospitals are having more difficulty justifying their health care costs.

- University hospitals have been relatively uninvolved in recent aggressive changes in the health delivery system: multihospital systems, shared services systems, HMOs, etc.
- By introducing the prospective-payment mechanism diagnosis related groups (DRGs), the federal government is trying to pare down hospital costs with interhospital competition. University hospitals, because they are teaching hospitals, often cannot easily cut out procedures and cannot be as competitive.
- University hospitals simply have had few reasons until recently to justify managing and governing themselves, outside of their governance by university trustees.

John Westerman, former executive director of the University of Minnesota Hospitals and Clinics, went to the heart of the situation:

> [The fundamental issue is to distinguish] between the continued existence of the university system and its performance of its basic educational mission, versus its continued ability to grow as a valuable social institution in a position of excellence and leadership.
>
> [Unfortunately the] usual and customary rigors of individual and academic unit performance review are strangely absent when it comes to how well the university operates a hospital. It's not that there is some sort of cover-up plot to not evaluate mission and performance, it's just that the right questions are never asked.... The question of how well university hospitals are managed must be deferred to the question of how they can be made manageable . . .

In discussing how to focus our research efforts in this area, we realized that no study of any topic would yield useful results unless we understood the governance (or policy-making) and management (or operational) structures of the institutions involved. The questions of finance, mission, and organizational relationships would have to wait until we understood better the matters of governance that seemed to be at the root of the hospitals' dilemma.

We cannot begin to understand the governance and management of university-owned hospitals until we identify what sets these hospitals apart from others. First of all, university-owned hospitals are different from other short-term, nonfederal, general hospitals in that they must balance patient care with teaching and research. Furthermore, university ownership makes them wholly owned operating divisions constrained by the interests and decisions of their parent university. Teaching status combined with university ownership means that the university hospitals' structure tends to mirror the academic divisions of the related medical school, and they tend to be staffed by clinicians who are part of the medical school and thus subject to influence by the medical school's administration. It is not teaching per se that distinguishes university hospitals but the degree or extensiveness of that commitment. Although approximately 1,300 hospitals are involved with some form of teaching, only 327 are considered primary teaching hospitals by the American Hospital Association; of those, 64 are actually owned by a university—20 by private universities and 44 by public universities.

The importance of university hospitals is demonstrated in their contribution being grossly disproportionate to their numbers. Although the 327 primary teaching hospitals constitute only 5.6 percent of all hospitals, they provided 40 percent of all charity care in 1980 [1]. Of these, the 64 university hospitals provided 10 million days of patient care and generated $5.5 billion in operating revenues in 1981. As the base hospitals for many of the 127 medical schools in the United States, teaching hospitals fund 75 percent of the costs of residency training. A disproportionate number of these hospitals provide the major source of primary care in financially depressed inner cities. Finally, advances in medical technology often originate with medical faculty, are first instituted in university hospitals, and sometimes remain available only within these hospitals. Clearly they perform a critical role in this nation's health system.

DEVELOPING THE INITIAL INVESTIGATIVE FRAMEWORK

As we defined the object of study, we encountered the first of many problems of definition: How to define what a university hospital organization is.

The university hospital as a physical plant can be defined with little disagreement, but defining it as an organization is more controversial, for important purposes are served by defining it in quite different ways. For example, the university hospital may be seen as:

— a distinct, separate entity

— a necessary part of an integrated teaching resource

— an important (and costly) component of a university

Even these statements do not catch the full flavor of the difference. Think of it this way: Is the hospital payroll part of the hospital or part of the university payroll department? And, most crucially, who decides? Does the university administration have a responsibility for deciding to centralize or decentralize payroll operations? Or is the decision to administer (or subcontract) payroll activities a hospital operating responsibility?

We chose an investigative framework that addresses such questions in a relatively neutral way. It rests on applications of open systems theory to the study of organizations, viewing the organization simultaneously as a distinct entity and as part of a larger entity. This dual view allows us to link both external and internal forces in the consideration of organizational phenomena. It also allows us to select among several starting points in studying organizations. We selected the starting point of studying a focal organization.

In considering external and internal forces, we recognized how complex and crucial the university hospital's environment is. At a university hospital, many environmental forces converge. It is a place in which the medical school faculty teach, provide care, and do research. It is a place to which the state, as the "owner" of state institutions, is likely to look for indigent care, for advanced tertiary care, and for medical innovation. It is a place which the parent university traditionally governs. While university hospitals have to be responsive to this ownership environment, they also have to respond to their competitive environment, which is made up of other health care professionals and tertiary care centers. What happens within these hospitals may frequently be attributable to environmental pressures. University hospitals are therefore wide-open systems whose rise and fall are intimately tied to the vicissitudes of their environments. Such vicissitudes reflect uncertainties involving huge stakes. No wonder that the two topics university presidents are rumored to talk about most are their college football teams and their university hospitals!

Our initial framework—viewing university hospitals as open systems—drew on the ideas of James Thompson, particularly on two key notions: (1) an organization such as a university hospital is open to its environment because it has no choice; and (2) such an organization constantly seeks to limit this openness in order to achieve a measure of efficiency [2]. Since this tension is present in every university hospital, a framework that recognizes it as a core truth has much to commend it.

The concept of environment is an important one in the study of organizations. It describes those influencing factors that are outside the boundaries of the focal organization (or individual), and are either uncontrollable or only partially controllable. It is often useful to describe an organization's environment by its members, that is, competitors, referring physicians, and the state legislature. Those members that are more significant in providing or restricting access to resources are described as part of the "task environment" [3].

Perhaps the most important characteristics of an organization's environment are those that have a direct impact on the organization. Whether the environment is simple or complex, stable or unstable, munificent or barren, whether resources are concentrated or dispersed, and whether members of the task environment accept the organization's needs and purposes—these describe environmental characteristics directly relevant to goal attainment and even survival of the particular organization [4].

Of these descriptive characteristics we make particular use of two: the degree of uncertainty that a university hospital faces in its environment, and the degree of dependence that the hospital has upon one or several members in its environment. Both of these are central to the understanding of university hospital behavior. As uncertainty increases, survival is more likely if those within the university hospital who can deal effectively with that uncertainty have the freedom and resources to do so. The dependence variable helps identify the key, or critical, members of the task environment: those who provide resources that cannot easily be replaced [5].

From these ideas we further developed the major underpinnings of the framework, as noted below:

— The study focus is the university *hospital,* not the health science complex, the university, or (in the case of state university hospitals) the state.
— The hospital is treated as a facility that can (and must) serve many interests, and that therefore can be seen as a part of the university organization, as a part of the academic health center organization, or as itself, a separate organization.
— Governance is in part a process of determining priority and balance among powerful, changing, and divergent interests.

These assumptions allowed us to consider important variations in where governance decisions are made (e.g., state level, university level, academic health center level, hospital level), and variations in how fully centralized the governance functions are at these levels. The assumptions also allowed us to isolate the factors that might properly lead decision makers in a university hospital to shift or reinforce the current location of governance functions.

The assumptions led us to a study framework that had three important components: (1) sources of pressures operating on the university hospital, (2) characterizations of the hospital itself, and (3) measures of outcome of performance.

In considering these components, we knew we needed a framework that took us outside the walls of the hospital. Our initial model was elemental (see figure 2.1).

It recognized three sets of variables, and also recognized the fact that the environment might influence outcomes directly as well as through the hospital. Once we saw the major outlines of the task, we refined this model (see figure 2.2).

Most significantly, we split "environment" into two types, loosely described as "outer" and "inner." The outer environment (left side of figure 2.2) reflects the marketplace, and includes political, economic, competitive, and regulatory pressures. The outer environment is shared with other community and teaching hospitals. The inner environment includes those who feel a sense of ownership of the hospital, and is thus specific to that particular hospital.

We also identified three types of management problems that plague university hospitals, though in differing degrees: (1) managing support services, (2) preventing financial vulnerability, and most importantly (3) setting the direction and managing the performance of patient care delivery. These issues are discussed beginning with chapter 8 of this volume.

FURTHER THEORETICAL PERSPECTIVES

Thompson's concepts clearly helped set the stage for our initial theoretical explanation of university hospitals. However, our theoretical considerations did not stop there; we incorporated additional perspectives during early stages of our investigations. The three models presented here provide lenses with which to view the phenomenon of university hospitals.

Resource-Dependence Perspective

University hospitals may essentially be viewed as a set of service activities that is highly dependent on the availability of resources. These resources may take many forms, such as patients, personnel, or reimbursement. To the extent that such resources are abundant, the hospital activities are stable and predictable. When resources are scarce, as in a highly competitive setting, the routine process of hospital activities is disrupted. From this perspective, resources dictate the type and structure of activities within a hospital. The hospital will be viable if it can structure itself in order to exploit resources.

This resource-dependence model is the simplest explanation of the plight of university hospitals: some university hospitals are more

Figure 2.1 General Research Model

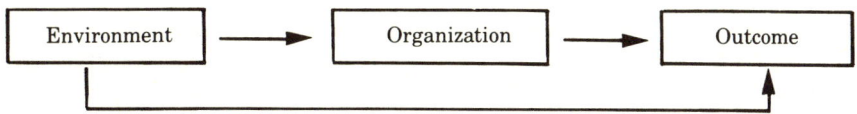

Figure 2.2 Delineated Research Model

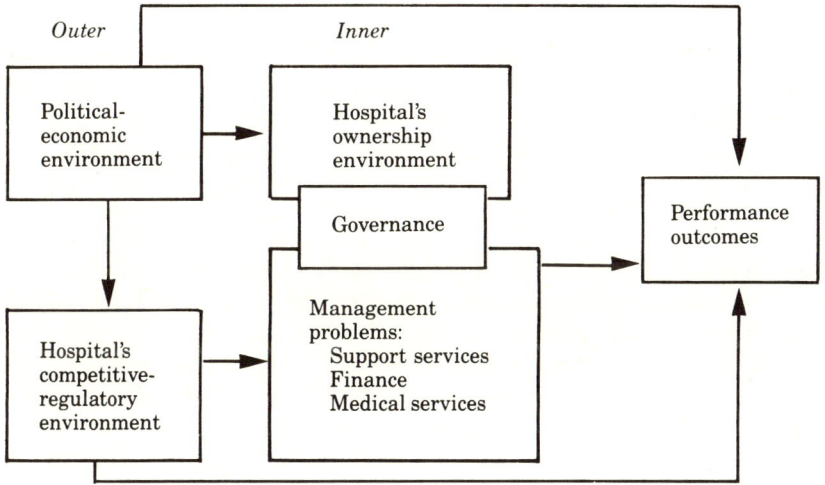

viable than others because their environmental resources are abundant [5]. Therefore, a resource-abundant environment helps a university hospital; a lack of resources hurts it. According to this model, it follows that an organization changes because it must adapt to changes in the amount and type of available resources in the environment. The model assumes that organizations are capable of continuous adaptation.

Obviously, all organizations need resources, but to describe this need as the sole raison d'être of university hospital structure and behavior would miss some of the intricacies of such a complex institution. So we sought additional explanations.

Population-Ecology Model

When we started our initial site visits of hospitals, we were struck by the amount of competition even in so-called resource-rich environments, and by the amount of "doom and gloom"—real fear of organizational demise—in a notable number of university hospitals. We were somewhat surprised at this, since university hospitals are generally seen as "megaloinstitutions" with unlimited resources and resourcefulness. Any rumor of financial distress is usually treated as just that—rumor. But the more we learned about university hospitals, the more we understood their fears. There was for us researchers the sense of discovery that the newly elected John F. Kennedy had when he remarked "the country's financial state under the previous Republican administration really *is* as bad as we claimed during our campaign."

The worries of university hospitals about survival may be justified less by resource scarcity (the resource-dependence explanation) than by the hospitals' incapacity to adjust to changes in resource availability (the population-ecology explanation). When new resources suddenly open up or old resources suddenly disappear, some university hospitals are not prepared to exploit changes swiftly and deftly.

The resource-dependence model outlined earlier indicated that organizations need resources, but did not indicate why some organizations are better able to attain them. The population-ecology model begins to provide some clues [6].

In brief, the population-ecology model says that within a class of organizations (such as university hospitals), any sudden changes may catch some short due to the inability to adapt quickly enough. Those organizations that adapt will survive; those whose adaptability is slowed by inertia, will fail. Adaptability is enhanced when the hospital has resources—that is, organizational slack—to cushion against sudden environmental shifts. Moreover, if such slack is liquid, as in the form of unencumbered reserve funds, it can be transformed quickly to help the hospital.

Organizational slack may also be viewed as something less liquid but just as effective. For example, university hospitals that enjoy a good reputation may be able to weather changes better, for these hospitals are often given special allowances—rate-setting regulations, reimbursement caps, capital expansion permits, etc. The population-ecology model views the environment as changing, and seeks to identify which type of organization will survive under the new condition. In this model the environment determines which type of organization will survive. As our study proceeded, we found this model of environmental determinism appealing but not fully satisfactory.

For example, the overall inefficiencies of some university hospitals, which may be considered an indicator of organizational inertia, are largely accepted as a by-product of the teaching and research missions of the hospital. The fact that these hospitals are not cost competitive does not seem to spell demise. Thus, state protection weakens the harsh predictions of environmental selection.

This protectedness causes the university hospital not to fit exactly into the population-ecology model, because that model works best for an organization in an intensely competitive and unprotected environment. Although the most recent thinking about population ecology acknowledges the presence of such protection, we considered a third perspective providing a view of university hospitals that clearly recognizes the importance of protectedness [7].

Protected-Organizations Perspective

Since the survival of university hospitals seems to be wholly explained neither by resource dependency nor by environmental selection, and since we acknowledge that university hospitals are open systems, then some unaccounted-for element in the environment must offer protectedness. The theories of Meyer and Rowan offer an explanation [8].

According to Meyer and Rowan, institutionalized products, services, techniques, policies, and programs (such as those commonly seen in hospitals) conform to institutionalized or societally expected rules, which may often conflict sharply with, and even work against, organizational efficiency. Therefore, enforcing efficiency at the expense of societal norms and expectations may very well erode societal support and legitimacy. The point here is simply this: state officials (who act in the capacity as "owners," see fig. 2.2) see their state-owned university hospital not only as a place for care, research, and teaching, but also as a symbol of state pride. These owners are not solely or overly concerned with efficiency per se. Rather, they take pride in "their" hospital's important medical breakthroughs, its quality of education and patient care, and its exemplary professional behavior—all of which are often antithetical to economic efficiency. Some university hospitals may in fact be forced by state regulations to be *in*efficient. For example, a surplus of funds at the end of any given fiscal year may mean that the state will automatically reduce its appropriation or subsidization for the hospital the following year. In sum, the viability of university hospitals is not necessarily dependent on efficiency except perhaps when the state particularly insists on it. This perspective suggests that university hospitals do not have to be commercially competitive in order to remain viable. Rather, university hospitals embody or reflect certain values of the state that may not necessarily dovetail with all-out efficiency.

As mentioned earlier, when population ecologists refer to organizational slack, they mean resources necessary for organizational survival. That is, organizations with greater slack are able to withstand longer periods of uncertainties and unanticipated misfortunes. We may view the protectiveness from the state as a form of organizational slack. This desire to protect probably stems from tradition, sentiment, perpetuation of a value system, and pride in the state institution. Despite the clear presence of a competitive market environment, the university hospital is not singularly immersed in that environment alone. Many university hospitals, by virtue of what they mean to their states, are also in a protected environment.

Of course, some environments are more protective or supportive than others. How protectiveness differs, and why, is inexorably linked to the characteristics of state ownership and is a continuing major theoretical and analytical focus of our study. For the moment, it is important to note that in varying degrees, officials in states view their university hospitals much as major stockholders view their heavily invested firms. The university hospital will not be allowed to die. But, unlike commercial firms which are made to be more sensitive to the vagaries and mercy of competitive pressures in the marketplace, the university hospital is a symbol—again, to varying degrees—of state pride and commitment. Its ability to compete is not necessarily of the utmost importance to state officials. Consequently, while the relative inefficiency prevents some university hospitals from being competitive in the market environment, the strong ownership environment protects them from failure. The protection given by the institutional environment provides a form of organizational slack or reserve which removes the university hospital from do-or-die competition.

In essence, university hospitals exist in multiple environments, and these environments are not necessarily compatible or consistent. Thus, the lack of a clear fit between the structure of the university hospital and its environment may in fact be a consequence of the need for the university hospital to be responsive to multiple and inconsistent environments. It is in this light that Weick's notion of "loose coupling" seems particularly relevant to our study [9]. That is, the university hospital cannot afford to be tightly linked and adapted to any single environment, given that the demands and available resources of the diverse environments are different, and that each environment is functionally important to the hospital.

Hence, to understand the university hospital requires an understanding of its multiple environments. As mentioned earlier, two of particular interest are the competitive and the ownership environments. The former deals with technical and market constraints. The latter deals with university-state constraints. Understanding the nature of both of these environments and their impacts illuminates the governance, management, and performance of state-owned university hospitals.

METHODOLOGY: DATA AND SOURCES

As we designed our study, we found that the richness and complexity of university hospitals could only be conveyed through the use of a variety of data sources. Accordingly, we secured information from diverse sources and drew heavily on prior work, notably the study of academic health center governance by the Association of Academic Health Centers, and the work done on university hospital governance by Robert Allison and Jeptha Dalston [10,11]. We used four basic data sources:

1. Published statistical data from the American Hospital Association for 1980, Association of American Medical Colleges (AAMC), the Census Bureau, and various states
2. Financial and operating data authorized by individual university hospitals and provided for 1979–81 by the Council of Teaching Hospitals, AAMC
3. Intensive field studies (a pilot) of 15 university hospitals—interviewees in this study included university regents, presidents, chief executive officers (CEOs) of hospitals, state legislators, clinical chiefs of staff, university administrative officials, hospital advisory board members, allied health personnel, and competitors
4. Primary data gathered from questionnaire survey responses by 52 of the 64 university-owned hospitals in the United States, public and private

We requested data from the universe of 64 university hospitals (20 private and 44 state owned), with an overall response rate of 86 percent (77 percent for state owned alone).

In particular, the field interviews and the more detailed data gathered during each visit proved invaluable. They helped frame the survey instrument, and provided explanatory detail of the linkage between performance outcomes and the variables that caused them. From these interviews, we began to see more clearly the complex interpenetration of operating and policy decision processes, and the remarkable variation in management and governance structures among university hospitals.

Nonrespondent Hospitals

University hospitals are scattered across the United States. We judged that state and regional differences, which we found to be critical, are adequately represented in our study. State-owned university hospitals are located in 35 states; respondents are distributed over 33 of these states, with Texas and Utah not represented. We judge that nonrespondents did not significantly affect our ability to generalize our results.

METHODOLOGY: DATA ANALYSIS

Data analysis was done primarily in three forms: correlations, scaling or indexing, and path analysis. All three are briefly described here.

Correlations

Correlation analysis describes the degree to which two variables move together (positive correlation), or in opposite directions (negative correlation). When a significance test is added, it is possible to determine how often such a correlation would be found by chance.

When a correlation is based on a small sample (say, 10 or 15), a single "outlier"—that is, a hospital very different from the majority on one of the two variables—can have a major influence on a correlation and its significance. Under such circumstances, we made it a rule to remove outliers in excess of four standard deviations from the mean. In this way we were able to inspect correlations not excessively influenced by a single observation.

Correlations are often used to strengthen the confidence that researchers have in the validity of a particular measure. One such example from our study will make this clear. We used a financial viability measure (chapters 3, 6, 7, and 8) that is the ratio of total operating revenues (less appropriations) to total operating expenses. Despite some weaknesses in this measure (see chapter 4), we believed it closely approximated the concept of viability, and we used correlations with other measures to validate this belief.

That is, if viability is defined as the ability of the state-owned university hospital to thrive independently (without appropriations) in the marketplace, we would expect that a viable hospital would be efficient. Such viability allows the hospital to be less reliant on external sponsorship and therefore relatively free of ownership or control by outside forces. Hence, viability should correlate in predictable ways with several variables, as in fact it does. Viability correlates positively with efficiency ($r = .53$), and correlates negatively with control of the university hospital by the state ($r = -.27$), by university regents ($r = -.19$), and by the medical school ($r = -.27$). The pattern of correlations and their expected directions help strengthen the confidence we have in the validity of this viability measure.

Scaling

As mentioned, we collected extensive data from multiple sources, some of which were longitudinal. Because we had so much data, we combined similar data into scales for manageability. By so doing, we moved from single-item variables to a composite made up of multiple items. Because concepts are more comprehensively represented by this composite, we are more confident in its reliability [12]. Assuming that a given set of data reflect a common underlying concept such as "market competition," we would assume that all data purporting to measure market competition are intercorrelated. The higher the intercorrelations, the more reliable will be the index.

A summary coefficient that tells the degree of intercorrelation among the composite variables in a given scale is Cronbach's alpha [13]. To the extent that Cronbach's alpha is high (e.g., over 0.70, with a range of 0.00–1.00), the scale is said to be reliable. Variables that do not contribute to high reliability—judged by their attenuating effect on alpha—are removed from a composite and would therefore not become part of that scale.

Once a composite is judged to be homogeneous (having an acceptable alpha), it is subjected to factor analysis [14]. The idea here is that a composite which purports to measure a common underlying concept will be shown by factor analysis to have a common underlying factor. Thus, a single-factor solution from factor analysis substantiates the homogeneity of variables chosen for a given scale. To put it another way, those variables share common variance.

When a scale has been judged reliable, scale scores can be assigned to each case. At that point, scales can be used in the same way as the individual variables are used in data analysis, that is, in correlations. Scale scores have a distribution just like single variable scores. Scale scores are based on the sum of scores from each of the composite variables in that scale, provided these variables are standardized—having the same mean (0) and standard deviation (1.0)—and coded in the appropriate direction. For example, in a "market competition" index, each composite variable is coded in a way consistent with the scoring of the "market competition" index. That is, a high score in the composite variable is in fact a high score in "market competition."

Path Analysis

We used path analysis (path coefficients) to estimate and compare the magnitudes of the effects of different variables on each other (e.g., impact of environmental variables on governance, management, and hospital viability) [15].

A path model (for example, those in chapters 6, 7, and 9) is essentially a sequential compilation of regression equations. These equations can be easily identified by first noting the number of dependent variables in the path model. Dependent variables are readily identifiable because they are always pointed to by single-headed arrows. At the other end of the arrow or path is the corresponding independent variable. Each path specifies the relationship between one independent variable and one dependent variable. As with most research, there are more independent variables than there are dependent variables. There are as many paths as there are independent variables, and a dependent variable in one particular regression equation may serve as an independent variable in another regression equation, as the above-mentioned path models will show.

This approach represents sequential regression of antecedent and dependent variables at various points in the model. The antecedent (independent) variables must be standardized, so that the beta or path coefficients in the regression equations are comparable and allow us to analyze the relative influence between coefficients. Each coefficient simply signifies how much effect an independent variable has on the dependent variable. And if there are other independent variables affecting the same dependent variable (i.e., other paths leading to that variable), the relative influence of each independent variable may be compared as in standard regression analysis [16].

A particular advantage of path analysis lies in its explicitness. All of the postulated relationships are diagramatically shown, often in one path model. The sequential chain of causal relationships, which is often cumbersome to describe, is picture explicit in a path diagram. A path model may also be seen as a diagram of a theory involving a complex set of causal relationships, whether real or hypothetical. The coefficients derived from regression analyses serve to confirm or substantiate the theory.

From a data analytic vantage point, path analysis allows us not only to assess the direct effect between each independent variable on a dependent variable, but also to calculate the indirect effect of an independent variable on a dependent variable through other variables along the path. As limitations are inherent in all data analytic techniques, path analysis faces the same limitations of regression analysis, above all that path analysis is recursive. That is, it is a unidirectional system that precludes the estimation of mutual causation between variables. But as with all model building in studies of this kind, the model aims to present a simplified reality, not an exact replication with all of its myriad complexities intact.

STUDY LIMITATIONS

This study of governance and management of university hospitals leaves several questions unanswered, or answered with less precision than we would like. There are four important limitations.

Limitations on Data Availability

Some data are very costly or nearly impossible to collect. Two examples are comparative data on the quality of medical care, and case-mix data. The absence of the former limits ability to measure an important dimension of performance. The absence of the latter makes it difficult to distinguish between resource allocations that produce a more expensive product (a more complex case mix) and those that are simply inefficient.

A second problem is simply missing data. Since there are only 64 university hospitals, the sample size is quite small for some multivariate data analytic techniques. Missing data can further exacerbate the small-sample-size problem and may undermine the confidence we have in some of the results.

We handled some of the problems by using data gained in the field study interviews; we handled others by using proxies. Nevertheless, missing data has been a constraint on this study. As a result, we exercised caution in how we interpreted our data.

Limitations of Data Reliability

In this study we had to choose between collecting specifically relevant data, or using available but less well-focused data that would potentially be incomparable. We compromised by doing both: constructing and disseminating a manageable survey, and making use of available data.

We also made hard choices in our survey selection. We could work for a high rate of return from a single respondent, or accept a lower return rate from three or more respondents. We chose the first option, and selected also the respondents from whom the fullest data could be secured—in this case, the hospital directors. Obviously, we then had to cope with a possible bias in their answers to questions that required judgment or opinions. We kept subjective questions to a minimum and asked questions potentially verifiable. We were also helped by our extensive field interviews, that gave us a relatively clear sense of what goes on in university hospitals.

A different kind of reliability problem arose from varying definitions of desired performance. In other words, the way one hospital defines its mission—its desired performance—may vary from another's definition, so we could not apply a single meaning to the performance data of both. For example, four university hospitals we studied had an exact zero net surplus in 1980. Obviously this cannot happen unless one starts with the necessity of having a net zero surplus, and then adjusts other figures to fulfill this objective.

One strength is worth noting. The data on all university hospitals come from three separate sources. Generally, data about the environment come from secondary and census data, data about the organization from the CSUH survey, and data about performance from the AAMC's Council of Teaching Hospitals (COTH) financial and general operating data. This minimizes the danger of overlooked autocorrelation—that is, of thinking we have discovered important truths in the relation between two variables, when in reality the relationship exists because the data for both variables come from the same source. This should strengthen confidence in the relations found across three independent data sets.

Limitations in Methodology

Even though substantially complete data were available from 52 of the 64 hospitals, the total population is still so small and varied that we could not avoid the "every university hospital is unique" problem. In such a population, there are too many possible explanations for phenomena and too few hospitals to test which explanations are true, or generalized to the entire population. In subsequent chapters, we will clearly point out the key areas in which this lack of statistical validity warrants a cautious interpretation of the findings.

Limitations of Cross-Sectional Analysis

In organizations, important actions often do not have immediate outcomes. For example, an expansion in scope of services does not immediately increase occupancy, nor does a change in leadership immediately improve performance. An historical study could have handled some of these lagged effects, but our cross-sectional study by its nature limited our ability to make confident predictions about causality. This problem was accentuated by our need to use data for the construction of performance indices that applied to the hospitals' fiscal year ending 1981, rather than in 1982 or 1983.

These four limitations are important in recognizing what the study could not do. The emphasis in this book, however, will not be to provide repeated qualifications, but to present as clearly as possible the findings of the study, and the data that support them.

REFERENCES

1. Schramm, C.J. The teaching hospital and the future role of state government. *New England Journal of Medicine* 308(1983):41–45.
2. Thompson, J.D. *Organizations in action.* New York: McGraw-Hill, 1967.
3. Dill, W.R. Environment as an influence on managerial autonomy. *Administrative Science Quarterly* 2(1958):409–43.
4. Aldrich, H.E. *Organizations and environment.* Englewood Cliffs, N.J: Prentice-Hall, Inc., 1979.
5. Pfeffer, J., and G. Salancik. *The external control of organizations: A resource-dependence perspective.* New York: Harper and Row, 1978.
6. Hannan, M.T., and J. Freeman. The population ecology of organizations. *American Journal of Sociology* 82(1977):929–64.
7. _____. Structural inertia and organizational change. *American Sociological Review* 49(1984):149–64.
8. Meyer, J.W., and B. Rowan. Institutionalized organizations: Formal structure as myth and ceremony. *American Journal of Sociology* 83(1977): 340–63.
9. Weick, K.E. Educational organizations as loosely coupled systems. *Administrative Science Quarterly* 21(1976):1–19.
10. Crispell, K.R., et al. *The organization and governance of academic health centers. Presentation of findings. Vol. 2.* Washington, D.C.: Association of Academic Health Centers, 1980.
11. Allison, R., and J. Dalston. Governance of university-owned teaching hospitals. *Inquiry* 19(1982):3–17.
12. Carmines, E.G., and R.A. Zeller. *Reliability and validity assessment.* Beverly Hills, Calif.: Sage Publications, 1979.

13. Cronbach, L.J. Coefficient alpha and the internal structure of tests. *Psychometrika* 16(1951):297–334.
14. Kim, J., and C.W. Mueller. *Factor analysis: Statistical methods and practical issues.* Beverly Hills, Calif.: Sage Publications, 1978.
15. Duncan, O.D. Path analysis: Sociological examples. *American Journal of Sociology* 72(1966):1–16.
16. Bohrnstedt, G.W., and D. Knoke. *Statistics for social data analysis.* Itasca, Ill.: F.E. Peacock, Publishers, Inc., 1982.

THREE

University Hospitals and Their Environment

What makes university hospitals distinct from other hospitals? Previous researchers have focused on various structural and environmental characteristics [1]. Butler and Bentley identified the cause in the link with the university and medical school [2]. Another group focused on the form of governance controlling university hospitals [3]. We have chosen to direct our attention not only to these individual factors but to the surrounding environment, thereby suggesting that the crucial distinction lies in the systematic relationship among elements in the environment, a university hospital's structural characteristics, and its ultimate performance.

The key words here are "systematic relationship." By examining a multitude of variables and correlating them one with another, we have been able to suggest a context within which a university hospital may be termed successful or viable, and to obtain a clearer picture of the external pressures and their appropriate internal responses.

This chapter explores the relationships between the university hospital's environment and its governance structure. In order to do this, we correlated four contextual variables with seven governance variables. Data for the contextual variables were obtained largely through census data and similar sources. Data for the governance variables were obtained through an individual questionnaire survey. The range of variables can best be seen by reviewing table 3.1. The remainder of this chapter discusses each of these variables in detail, as well as the results of the statistical correlations between the variables in the two columns.

Contextual Variable #1: Market and Political Environment

Although university hospitals are influenced by numerous environmental forces (for example, DRGs), they are individually influenced by economic forces in their respective state markets and by the political forces unique to each state. We constructed the market and political environment indexes from these variables, according to the method of scaling described in chapter 2:

Market index
— Per capita personal income, average per state resident
— Urbanization (percent residents living in standard metropolitan statistical areas over 50,000)
— Number of M.D. specialists in patient care practice per 100,000 residents

Political index
— Political culture (progressivism or proactive, progovernment values) [4,5].
— Legislative innovation (months required to pass model legislation) [6,7,8,9].
— Interparty competition (extent of two-party versus one-party control) [10].

The market index is made up of three highly intercorrelated variables. This means that a highly urbanized state is likely to be relatively wealthy and to have a high ratio of physician specialists to the state's population. And since urbanization is a proxy for the existence of regional medical centers, a state scoring high on this index is likely to have many physician specialists practicing in well-equipped regional medical centers. Most importantly, these factors mean high market competition for university-owned hospitals.

We used the three political index variables together with the market index variables for several reasons. These same urbanized, wealthy states are likely to be characterized by a "progressive" or "proactive" political culture and a political system which is, due to interparty competition, responsive to these values. Consequently, the legislature tends to be innovative—as measured by the speed with which pro-

Table 3.1 Contextual and Governance Variables Used

Contextual Variables	Governance Variables
Environment Market and political index (environment) Ownership (public vs. private) Source of net patient revenues (state appropriations) *Organizational structure* Size (number of beds)	Type of board Size of board Board focus: internal/external Board emphasis on governance/management Board proactivity Key group decision making Board effectiveness

gressive legislation is passed. The strong association between the market and political indexes (correlation coefficient = 0.76) justifies treating both indexes as a measure of the state environment.

We used data from 33 states for political indexes to define three types of statewide environments in which university hospitals find themselves. The first type has the highest overall score in state proactivism and competitiveness, and the third type the lowest. It is possible that some states are extremely proactive, but only moderately competitive, or some other combination. By means of cluster analysis, we sorted out states into three general clusters, as shown in table 3.2.

Table 3.2 Political and Economic Environment of University Hospitals

Group I High Proactive/ Competitive States	Group II Proactive/ Competitive States	Group III Low Proactive/ Competitive States
Illinois	Minnesota	Mississippi
New York	Ohio	N. Carolina
Washington	Pennsylvania	W. Virginia
California	Indiana	Virginia
Massachusetts	Nebraska	Georgia
Maryland	Wisconsin	Louisiana
Connecticut	Iowa	Arkansas
New Jersey	Oregon	Missouri
Colorado	Kansas	Kentucky
Michigan	Arizona	S. Carolina
		Alabama
		Florida
		Tennessee

We drew three major conclusions from the data in table 3.2. First, states south of the Mason-Dixon line, or on its border, form a definite subtype (group III) both economically and politically. Second, groups I and II are mostly northern states, and have the most stringent forms of rate regulation. Third, the environment of northern and western states is more constraining to university hospitals than that of southern states because those in the north face a combination of both high market competition and stringent regulation from state governments.

For example, the most challenging environment might be a university hospital in a northeastern state having many urban centers with excellent medical centers and a high ratio of physician specialists. This hospital faces severe market constraints, and is less likely to receive referrals from areas outside the university hospital's immediate service area. In addition, its state government is more likely to have stringent certificate-of-need laws and hospital rate regulation. Yet despite these constraints, a hospital in such a state is also quite likely to be protected by the state, as later chapters will show.

Contextual Variables #2 and #4: Ownership and Size

The variables ownership and size are easily described and are both shown together in table 3.3. In this study there were 34 public and 18 private university-owned hospitals. Size is measured by the number of beds staffed in 1981. The median size for all 52 hospitals is 545 beds.

Contextual Variable #3: State Appropriations

The third contextual variable is state appropriations as a percent of the university hospital's total operating revenues. Table 3.4 shows data from the Council of Teaching Hospitals, giving all the sources of support (state and others) for the 29 university hospitals included in their data base for the fiscal year 1982.

Of the 52 hospitals included in our study, 19 receive no appropriation and 33 receive some appropriation. The proportion of net patient revenue from appropriations for those receiving any appropriation ranges from a low of 1 percent to a high of 44 percent. Those university hospitals receiving the highest levels appear to be newer, as are their medical schools. Not all state university-owned hospitals receive a state appropriation, and some private university-owned hospitals do receive an appropriation—most notably in Pennsylvania. Hence, public ownership and appropriations are not synonymous, and both may be used as measures of a university hospital's dependence upon the state.

Table 3.3 Ownership and Size of University Hospitals

Public		Private	
Name (N = 34)	Beds 1981	Name (N = 18)	Beds 1981
Iowa	1028	NYU	682
Talmadge (Ga.)	938	Rochester	722
Michigan	889	Chicago	719
Alabama	804	Jefferson	687
Maryland	729	Pennsylvania	654
Minnesota	705	Stanford	689
Virginia	697	Vanderbilt	581
Illinois	689	Cincinnati	557
UCLA	685	Hannemann	542
Washington	646	Temple	540
Indiana	594	Emory	636
Kansas	584	Loma Linda	528
Mississippi	558	Geo. Wash. U.	512
Wisconsin	548	Georgetown	501
UCSF	544	McGaw	495
UMDNJ (N.J.)	536	CW Long (Emory)	470
LSU	528	Med. Coll. Pa.	385
N. Carolina	527	St. Louis	325
S. Carolina	458	Average =	568
Kentucky	455		
Florida	452		
W. Virginia	452		
Talmadge (Ga.)	427		
Missouri	426		
Oregon	401		
UC Davis	401		
Colorado	393		
S. Alabama	380		
Arkansas	355		
Hershey (Pa.)	331		
Massachusetts	309		
Nebraska	287		
Arizona	243		
Connecticut	216		
Average =	536		

Table 3.4 Sources of University Hospital Net Patient Revenue for Fiscal Year Ending 1982 (in Percents)

	Public (N = 19)	Private (N = 10)
Private sources*	40.2	43.4
Medicare	25.1	29.6
Medicaid	14.5	10.8
Other sources	6.9	10.3
State appropriations	13.3	5.9

*Blue Cross, commercial insurance, self-payors.

For the state university-owned hospitals in our survey, the average appropriation was 17.3 percent.

Governance Variable #1: Type of Board

In our study, we asked respondents to identify the individual or group that in fact governed or made decisions about the hospital, that is, the true or operational governing board as opposed to a figurehead governing body. Although 40 hospitals indicated they had a separate board for the hospital, only 14 identified this board as the operational board. Table 3.5 shows the responses.

In order to understand the implications of these responses, it helps to understand something of the governance history of a university hospital. Initially, this hospital is typically governed by the university's trustees (usually of public universities) or the medical school dean (usually of private universities). As it grows, its first change in governance is to create a hospital board to oversee the medical staff and meet accreditation criteria in regard to the medical staff. Often these boards begin with little authority in areas other than approving appointments to the medical staff. However, over time these essentially advisory groups gain experience and credibility and are given increasing authority. Hence, the data in table 3.5 portray a dynamic process of change over time.

A similar study by the Association of Academic Health Centers (AAHC) in 1978–79 produced results different from ours. In the AAHC study, 75 percent of the university hospitals were governed by the university's trustees—either directly by them or by one of their subcommittees. Comparable data from table 3.5 indicate that only 54 percent of university hospitals are governed by groups outside of and above the medical center. Two factors may account for this. First is the dynamic process that we identified above. Second, respondents in the AAHC study were not asked to distinguish between "real operating" and "merely formal" groups.

It is clear from table 3.5 that no dominant form of governance has emerged at this time. The important point for research is to identify what environmental and structural factors are associated with each type of governance.

Governance Variable #2: Size of Board

In any type of organization, the size of the governing board is believed by some researchers to be related to organization size (with larger organizations having larger boards) and environment dependency (greater dependency requiring larger boards) [11]. According to these theories, an organization needing to woo outside regulators or sources of capital would need a larger board, one with representatives from the key targeted agencies of that regulation or capital [12,13]. Conversely, a board stressing internal administration would tend to be smaller and composed of insiders.

A series of studies on community hospitals verifies this ownership-size-environmental-dependency link. Ownership affects environmental dependence in that privately owned hospitals are more likely to seek capital funds and operating subsidies from private donors and stock offerings, but publicly owned hospitals are more likely to seek these funds through governmental sources. Hence, Elling and Halebsky found that ownership per se influenced the extent to which hospitals sought community support as contrasted to governmental support [14]. Pfeffer likewise found that hospitals stressing linkages to their environment had larger boards and more outsiders on their boards than hospitals that stressed internal administration. Hospitals

Table 3.5 Type of Operational Board

	Frequency	%
Statewide body	1	2
University president/chancellor	2	4
University regents/trustees	15	29
Subcommittee of regents/trustees	10	19
Academic health center board	5	10
Hospital board	14	26
Internal hospital committee	5	10
	52	100

having boards of the optimal size and composition tended to grow more than other boards [15].

In contrast to community hospitals, university hospitals have apparently not sought as many members from the outside environment. Among the university hospitals in our study (table 3.6), governing bodies range in size from 5 to 50 members. The average-size board has 15 members, and half of all boards have from 6 to 15 members. The average board has 59 percent of its members drawn from outside, that is, not officials of the university or state agencies. One-fourth of the boards have no external members. These data indicate that university hospitals apparently have not stressed the function of linking to their environment.

Governance Variable #3: Internal or External Focus

As discussed earlier, an important characteristic of boards is their orientation toward internal administration, or toward elements in the external environment crucial to the hospital's interests. Table 3.7 shows how different boards function. The first two response categories are external in orientation and the last two are internal. Among the respondents, 59 percent are oriented internally and 41 percent externally. These results are consistent with earlier studies on size and composition of boards.

The data reported in table 3.7 indicate the function in which a board is most effective. However, most boards probably perform all of these functions in varying proportions. There is no simple link between composition and function: external board members do not necessarily focus on the external linkage function and internal members on administration.

A trustee on a board has a legal and an ethical responsibility to

Table 3.6 Size of University Hospital Operational Boards

Numbers of Members	Boards in Size Category	
	Frequency	%
1–5	9	17
6–10	15	28
11–15	10	19
16–20	9	17
21–30	6	11
31–50	5	9

Table 3.7 Board Focus

	Frequency	%
External		
Provides buffer, linkage with environment, state, university and medical school administration and other "owners"	17	33
Helps obtain sources and approvals from regulatory groups, reimbursers, philanthropists, etc.	4	8
Internal		
Sets directions through planning, monitoring	16	31
Helps manage the hospital; quality monitoring	14	28
	51	100

make decisions based on the best interest of the owners—not based on the trustee's relationship to some external organization or internal constituency. Therefore, a board needs good advocates more than equal representation of strategic constituencies [16]. Consequently, if a board is meeting this ideal, there would be no necessary correspondence between its composition and function.

Governance Variable #4: Emphasis on Governance or Management

In a related question, we asked each board to define itself by assessing the relative emphasis it gives to policymaking, which is clearly a governance function, and to operational management, which is not.

There is no consensual definition of "governance," but most definitions view governance and management as a continuum: governance emphasizes matters of more strategic, long-range importance affecting the entire organization, and management stresses implementation and narrower, short-term (even day-to-day) tactical matters. In effect, we asked how boards function in order to find out how they define governance.

The results of this question (table 3.8) showed that there is no more consensus among the respondents of our study than among views expressed in the literature. The respondents are split among the two polar extremes of governance and management and the midpoint

Table 3.8 Relative Emphasis of Board on Governance or Management

	Frequency	%
Strategic long-range, policy-type governance matters	17	33
Approximately equal governance and management matters	15	29
Operational, short-range, procedural management matters	20	38
	52	100

which includes equal proportions of both. The real usefulness of such a measure, however, is in its correlation with other attributes of a particular university hospital that provide indications associated with a given view of governance. Nevertheless, these results do indicate that a number of boards seem to be functioning beyond the areas typically assigned to boards.

Governance Variable #5: Board Proactivity

A great deal is known of the actual decision-making role of directors of for-profit corporations, but little is known about this role in nonprofit organizations like university hospitals. In general, most for-profit major corporation boards have a sizeable proportion of members who are corporate officers, and the board chairman and chief executive officer tend to lead, if not dominate, their board [17]. Indeed, Marris and Wood believe these two corporate employees are so emancipated from control by the real owners—stockholders—that the former lead their corporations in directions contrary to the best interests of the true owners [18,19]. Directors of nonprofit corporations have as much power, but for different reasons: a recent study of trustees of nonprofit organizations found that typically only the executive director of an organization has board membership, but that these boards nonetheless typically avoid policy discussions and accept the de facto decisions of the executive director [20].

Other studies suggest that hospital board directors have less independence and less direct power than directors of the above-mentioned organizations, but evidence of the proactivity of the university hospital board is mixed at best. Kovner found in a study of large hospitals in two Eastern states that their board members were much more independent of hospital directors, and that board members felt they were involved in setting goals, strategies, and policies [21]. Terrill found that one-third of the university hospitals in his study were directly governed by the university's board, and that one-fourth of the hospitals' chief executive officers were excluded from meetings of the university's board [22].

Table 3.9 shows the measure of board proactivity, or initiative, used in our study. Respondents were asked to indicate the statement that comprised the best description for their hospital.

Results indicate that university hospital boards are typically passive rather than proactive. In this respect, they are in reality closer to the corporate and nonprofit boards than to the idealized role set for them in the normative literature within the industry. In fact, university hospital boards seem to act like visitors deferring to the initiative and expertise of insiders, rather than acting like proactive trustees who closely monitor hospital activities and initiate changes. However, unlike the data concerning the internal-external focus (table 3.4) and governance-management dimensions of board function (table 3.5), the data in table 3.9 are unequivocal: university hospital boards, whether by choice or by force, tend toward passivity.

Governance Variable #6: Key Group Decision Making

In order to measure further the power or influence of eight key decision-making groups and officials, we asked the hospital CEO to record how much influence each key group would have over 14 governance-management decisions. The responses are shown in table 3.10. The varying verbal responses for a given decision (shown in the rows in that

Table 3.9 Board Proactivity

	Frequency	%
Typically endorses proposals referred to them	27	52
Creatively reacts to proposals of university and hospital officials	15	29
Works collaboratively with university and hospital officials in developing plans and controlling the decision process	9	17
Initiates plans-proposals and influences decisions about them	1	2
	52	100

Table 3.10 Influence of Key Groups

Key Decisions	Key Groups (Decision Makers)						
	State	Trustees	Hospital Board	University Officials	V.P. for Health	Medical School Administrators	Clinical Chiefs	Hospital Administrators
1. Choose and/or appoint a new hospital CEO	0.4	8.4	11.7	17.8	21.5	15.9	16.3	7.8
2. Reorganization at the governance level to give substantial autonomy to the university hospital	6.8	20.0	9.5	19.1	12.8	9.0	8.5	12.4
3. Reorganization of hospital management (e.g., decentralization) to place accountability with second level manager	0.3	1.7	5.8	8.9	13.6	7.4	10.5	51.8
4. Expanding or contracting scope of medical services (e.g., trauma center)	2.5	5.5	9.0	9.1	14.8	14.1	21.6	23.4
5. Allocations of space within the hospital	—	0.2	2.2	3.7	16.5	14.6	22.0	40.7

6. Future directions, and emphasis on, clinical research	0.6	2.5	3.6	9.1	13.6	24.3	30.5	15.8
7. Fund-raising (philanthropic)	0.1	11.4	10.6	22.2	16.3	11.2	11.7	16.4
8. Personnel policies and procedures	7.6	9.8	6.2	23.6	12.9	7.7	5.2	25.1
9. Operating budget allocations	5.4	8.9	10.1	12.9	14.7	9.3	10.4	28.4
10. Decisions on capital budget allocations	6.3	9.7	9.8	12.9	12.5	8.5	12.2	26.2
11. Decisions on amount and sources of capital financing (e.g., borrowing)	8.3	19.3	10.1	20.9	12.5	4.3	3.0	18.0
12. Determining who is appointed, and with what privileges, to the medical staff	—	6.3	11.2	4.3	10.1	20.2	35.6	12.3
13. How staff members are paid	4.5	3.9	3.1	8.7	12.6	15.8	16.9	32.8
14. Bed allocations by service	0.8	1.2	3.6	2.2	11.3	15.3	27.7	36.2

table) were standardized so that the total for all decision makers was 100. This standardization made it possible to compare the influence of the eight groups of decision makers while preserving their relative influence on any particular decision. The eight decision groups columns comprise the bureaucratic hierarchy in a university hospital, ranging from state officials down to hospital administrators. We also compared hospitals for degree of centralization by calculating a weighted-average score for all decisions and decision-making levels, that is, state level is level 8, trustees are level 7, and so on. We calculated dispersion (how many groups were involved) using a Gini-index measure, which provided a numerical score summarizing how many levels and officials are involved in decision making. For example, this matrix has 132 cells, each cell indicating that one decision-making official or group is influential in one decision. Entries in many cells indicate greater diffusion or participation in decision making than if entries occur in only a few cells. A high index score indicates great dispersion, and conversely a low score indicates more oligarchical decision making—that is, a concentration of power or control in one area.

The data in table 3.10 have a high degree of face validity. For example, the hospital administrator is especially strong in allocating hospital space and beds and in administrative reorganization, and weak in decisions to appoint a new hospital administrator and decisions normally the preserve of the medical staff. Similarly, the clinical chiefs and medical school administration are strong in clinical matters; state officials and university trustees are strong in reorganizing governance and in capital funding decisions. Overall, the results seem plausible and credible.

Hospital administrators view themselves as being the most influential decision maker in 8 of the 14 decisions, the chiefs and university officials each in 2 decisions, and the trustees and vice-president for health services each in 1 decision. Interestingly enough, they did not see the state officials, the hospital board, and medical school administration as being the most powerful influence in any decision. Overall the picture presented tends toward selective decentralization and diffusion of influence. The real usefulness of the data, however, is in their association with environmental, structural, and performance measures.

Governance Variable #7: Board Effectiveness

The final structural variable measures board effectiveness. The results (table 3.11) show a clear central tendency (toward the middle) in the

Table 3.11 Board Effectiveness

	Frequency	%
Highly effective	8	15
Effective	16	31
Mixed, varies by issue and over time	20	39
Ineffective	8	15
	52	100

distribution. Again, the usefulness of this measure depends on its association with other measures.

We have summarized the four contextual variables and the seven governance-structure variables individually. Now we can begin to match and compare the relevant variables between the two groups, in order to see the overall relationship between context and governance structure.

Environment (Market and Political Indexes) and Governance Structure

Of the seven variables characterizing governance structures, only two—board focus (table 3.7) and board proactivity (table 3.9)—were associated with the environmental variables (market competition and political proactivity, table 3.2).

First, in the comparison of environment with board orientation table 3.12 shows hospitals with the greater external orientation are found in group I—those having the greatest market competition and the most proactive state government.

One interpretation of these data is that a more dynamic and constraining environment, such as for group I, requires greater external orientation; conversely, an internal orientation is workable for a more stable, benevolent environment as in group III. Group II, as expected, has a structure midway between groups I and III.

Second is the comparison of environment with board proactivity. Table 3.13 shows that group I hospitals have the most proactive boards, and group II hospitals the least proactive boards. High proactivity combines the boards that initiate proposals with those who work collaboratively with hospital officials to develop board proposals. Low proactivity combines the scale categories of creatively reacting to management proposals and passively endorsing management's proposals.

Table 3.12 University Hospital Environment and Board Orientation

Board Orientation	Environment		
	% Group I High Competition, Proactive ($N = 17$)	% Group II ($N = 15$)	% Group III Low Competition, Not Proactive ($N = 17$)
External linkage function emphasized	76	60	35
Internal administrative function emphasized	23	40	65

Note: Chi square = 9.957, D.F. = 2, and Sig. = .05.

The interpretation offered for proactivity's relationship with environment is similar to that of orientation's relationship to environment. Boards for group I hospitals function primarily to link the hospital to its dynamic and challenging environment. In such an environment, they have a greater need to take initiatives. What remains unclear is the juxtaposition of groups II and III—the apparent fact that boards in the less dynamic, more benign group II environment are less proactive than boards in group III. This suggests the presence of confounding influences, or variables that were not included in this associational analysis, affecting the relationship.

Ownership and Governance Structure

The second contextual variable, that of ownership (public and private, table 3.3), was correlated with three of the seven governance structure

Table 3.13 University Hospital Environment and Board Proactivity

Proactivity	Environment		
	% Group I ($N = 17$)	% Group II ($N = 15$)	% Group III ($N = 18$)
High: initiates or collaborates	67	27	50
Low: reacts or endorses	35	73	50

Note: Chi square = 4.66, D.F. = 2, and Sig. = .0971.

measures—board function, centralization, power dispersion—and size. First, ownership has a substantive implication for board function. As table 3.14 shows, public hospital boards are approximately equally divided between external and internal emphasis. By contrast, private hospital boards clearly stress the role of external linkage—leaving internal administration to university and hospital officials.

The explanation for this is simple. Private universities depend on philanthropy for their operating subsidy; therefore their board members are selected at least in part for their ability to obtain needed funds. Moreover, private universities have the freedom to select board members on the basis of their expertise and environmental connections rather than their official position within the ownership hierarchy, as in public universities. Contrast this situation with that of public hospitals, which are subsidized by the state. Their boards are concerned with monitoring the hospital's stewardship of those state funds, and are therefore more internally focused. The lack of a dominant focus among the public hospitals is perhaps caused by the wide variation in the size of appropriation among public hospitals—a topic we will address in chapter 5.

University hospital ownership can also be compared with the centralization variable originally introduced in table 3.10. Most public hospitals are centralized and almost all private hospitals decentralized as measured by the centralization variable (see table 3.15).

This measure, as explained earlier, looks at the relative power that various groups of decision makers have in governance decisions. A "centralized" hospital is one in which higher levels exercise more power in governance; conversely in a "decentralized" hospital the power is diffused through lower levels. For this analysis, we dichotomized a range of scores on governance-related decisions (table 3.10) into centralized and decentralized categories, and analyzed them according to whether they were publicly or privately funded.

Table 3.14 University Hospital Ownership and Board Function

Board Function	Ownership	
	% Public ($N = 33$)	% Private ($N = 18$)
External linkage function emphasized	45	83
Internal administrative function emphasized	55	17

Note: Chi square = 6.8994, D.F. = 1, and Sig. = .0086.

Table 3.15 University Hospital Ownership and Centralization of Governance

Centralization of Power	Ownership	
	% Public (N = 33)	% Private (N = 18)
Centralized	55	17
Decentralized	45	83

Note: Chi square = 6.9, D.F. = 1, and Sig. = .01.

The ownership variable is strongly related to the dispersal of power—that is, how many major coalitions or official bodies are influential in decision making. In public hospitals, a large number of groups influence decisions, compared to relatively few groups in private hospitals (see table 3.16). One explanation for this is that philanthropic subsidies to private hospitals come with fewer strings attached, so university officials need be less involved in monitoring and controlling how funds are spent; in public hospitals, taxed-based subsidies tend to flow downward through successive layers of the government bureaucracy.

In viewing the last two variables, it is important to note that it is not philanthropy per se nor appropriations per se that influence either centralization or dispersion within governance. The real variable is control, which varies depending on who owns the hospital and who is doing the controlling. A state's citizens theoretically own their public university, but clearly there is no practical way for them to do so. In reality, public universities are controlled by state officials and members of the university's board. As the legal agents of the citizens, they control the tax-based subsidies to the university and in most cases its hospital. Every official in this legal-financial hierarchy—from state

Table 3.16 Ownership and Dispersion of Influence in Governance

Dispersion of power	Ownership	
	% Public (N = 34)	% Private (N = 18)
High (dispersed)	62	28
Low (focused)	38	72

Note: Chi square = 5.44, D.F. = 1, and Sig. = 0.197.

government through the university to its hospital—has potential leverage over the hospital's affairs. This is virtually a prescription for both centralization and diffusion of control.

By contrast, there are in fact seldom any true "owners" of private universities. If founded by a church (as many were), the financial and organizational ties have in many cases become attenuated or broken. If founded by a group of prominent citizens, they have long since died and been replaced by a self-perpetuating board. Although most are operated to benefit the public and are not-for-profit in form, they have never been owned by the public at large, nor been directly accountable to it. They are relatively independent of the public, and in need primarily of tuition-paying students, research funds, and philanthropic donations from alumni and other small segments of the public. In effect they are much closer to the Fortune 500-type corporation that is well insulated from control by the ultimate and true owners, the stockholders. Those providing financial resources in the form of tuition, research funds, and gifts typically exert little or no direct influence in governing board membership and governance decisions. Their boards thus are free to seek members with a desirable expertise or linkage with the external environment rather than those who merely hold a certain position within the university or have ties to its owners.

In private universities, the net result of these weak ties to the ultimate owners is decentralized governance focused within the university and health center, where power is based on access to information and expertise in operations. In the more bureaucratic public universities, the net result is a stronger tie to the owners, and a power based on legitimate claims made by owners.

Size and Governance Structure

Size (table 3.3) is not strongly related to any of the governance structure variables. The most likely reason for this is the absence of sufficient variation in size: most university hospitals are relatively large.

Appropriation and Governance Structure

We were able to contrast the third contextual variable, appropriation, with six governance structure variables: board age, board function, board proactivity, power dispersal in decision making, centralization of decision making, and board effectiveness. Appropriation is a measure of the hospital's dependence on the state and is conceptually distinguishable from state ownership per se. In this analysis, we dichotomized the range of scores for size of appropriation into "some" and "none" groupings. Six of the nine variables tested against appropriations were associated at the $p < .10$ significance level, which is significant.

First, we looked at appropriation and board age. As table 3.17 shows, hospitals receiving no appropriation tend to have "younger" boards. Since hospitals founded in recent years tend to have higher state appropriations, the most likely explanation for this apparent contradiction is that younger boards are not necessarily associated with new hospitals. Another factor is involved: hospitals not receiving an appropriation have the flexibility to change their governance structure more often, creating new boards to replace the prior, older system of control by the university's board of trustees.

Second, we looked at appropriation and board function (table 3.18). The absence of an appropriation is associated with an external board orientation, that is, the board focuses on external linkages and leaves management to hospital administrative officials. However, for hospitals receiving some appropriation the reverse relationship is much weaker, in other words, there is only a slight tendency for the board to focus on internal administration.

Table 3.17 University Hospital Appropriation and Board Age

	Appropriation	
Board Age	% None (N = 19)	% Some (N = 30)
Young	68	43
Old	32	57

Note: Chi square = 2.94, D.F. = 1, and Sig. = .08.

Table 3.18 Dependence on Appropriation and Board Function

	Appropriation	
Board Function	% None (N = 19)	% Some (N = 32)
External linkage	79	47
Internal administration	21	53

Note: Chi square = 5.06, D.F. = 1, and Sig. = .02.

The most likely explanation for the above relationship is that the absence of a tax subsidy is offset by philanthropic donations obtainable from the external environment through board activity. Secondly, most philanthropic donations—even those earmarked for a specific purpose—do not give the donor any rights to monitor continually and control the officials running the recipient organization. In contrast, tax monies have strings attached in the form of layers of government officials having the right to monitor and control expenditures. In fact these controls can go far beyond merely overseeing the funds provided by the state. Thirdly, state appropriations and philanthropy have historically been alternative rather than simultaneous sources of income, so very few state-owned university hospitals have had sizeable fund-raising drives. Their boards focus on coordinating the various university units and external payers and regulators involved in operations. Indeed, most of their board members are picked for their linkages with and expertise in these units. A related fact is that potential donors are reluctant to give to something their taxes are already subsidizing. But as state and federal financing gets tighter for all hospitals, state university-owned hospitals may be forced to seek more donated funds, in which case they may change their board composition accordingly.

Third, we looked at appropriation and board proactivity (table 3.19). Hospitals that receive no appropriation have boards more proactive than those receiving an appropriation. The explanation for this is a "chicken and egg" problem: we might conjecture that a more financially self-sufficient hospital got that way because it began with a proactive board. On the other hand, not having access to state subsidies may have forced the board to become proactive to remain financially viable. The statistical associations clearly show the strong relationship between a board's sole financial responsibility for hospital operations and board initiatives in fulfilling those responsibilities.

The fourth comparison is appropriations with dispersion of power in governance decision making (table 3.20). Because state appropria-

Table 3.19 Dependence on Appropriations and Board Proactivity

Proactivity	Appropriation	
	% None ($N = 19$)	% Some ($N = 33$)
Low (endorses/reacts)	32	64
High (initiates or collaborates)	68	36

Note: Chi square = 4.96, D.F. = 1, and Sig. = .03.

tions pass through the university, they give power to various university vice-presidents over functional departments, and thus tend to disperse influence over hospital governance. Even though appropriations comprise only 17 percent of the net patient revenues for the average state-owned university hospital in our study, they provide the rationale and leverage for university officials to become involved in the hospital's governance decisions. Rightly or wrongly this form of financial dependence, unlike any other form (e.g., patient reimbursement), expands the direct involvement of nonhospital officials in the hospital's governance decisions.

The fifth comparison is appropriations with centralization of governance decision making (table 3.21), which is probably strongly related to the dispersion factor just discussed. Appropriations tend to increase centralization of decision making. This is most likely a concomitant of dispersion, because by definition the individuals introduced into decision making as a consequence of controlling appropriations are at a higher level in the decision hierarchy.

The sixth and final comparison, appropriations with board effec-

Table 3.20 Dependence on Appropriations and Dispersion of Power in Governance Decision Making

Dispersion of Power	Appropriation	
	% None ($N = 19$)	% Some ($N = 33$)
Low	74	36
High	26	64

Note: Chi square = 6.72, D.F. = 1, and Sig. = .01.

Table 3.21 Dependence on Appropriation and Centralization of Governance Decision Making

Centralization of Power	Appropriation	
	% None ($N = 19$)	% Some ($N = 33$)
Centralization	21	67
Decentralization	79	33

Note: Chi square = 10.04, D.F. = 3, and Sig. = .001.

tiveness (table 3.22), shows that appropriations tend to make boards less effective. State appropriations are associated with greater dispersion and centralization of governance decision making, board passivity, and a primary emphasis on internal administration; those hospitals receiving an appropriation have operating boards considered less effective by the hospital CEO than those not receiving any appropriation. Of course, an alternative interpretation is possible: all these characteristics would occur if a nonviable university hospital with no state appropriation were placed in internal receivership by the university in an attempt to rescue it from financial disaster. However, based on our field interviews and the preponderance of findings reported herein, the first explanation seems more plausible.

Summary of All Comparisons: Contextual and Governance

Hospitals are governed by seven types of groups, with most being governed by either the university trustees or a separate hospital board. The typical board has 15 members of whom about 60 percent are from outside the hospital, university, or state in the case of public hospitals. Due to the wide variation, average board age is not a meaningful statistic to summarize the universe of university hospitals. About 40 percent of boards stress the function of linking the hospital to its external environment with 60 percent focusing on internal administration. There is no central tendency in terms of how the universe of boards gives stress to varying proportions of management versus governance.

Of the four contextual variables correlated with the governance structure variables, only size is unrelated to any governance measure. The measure combining political and economic environments was related to two measures of structure. States having a proactive government and competitive market are associated with externally oriented,

Table 3.22 Dependence on Appropriations and Board Effectiveness

Board Effectiveness	Appropriations	
	% None (N = 19)	% Some (N = 33)
Highly effective	21	12
Effective	42	24
Mixed/by issue	37	39
Ineffective	0	24

Note: Chi square = 6.5, D.F. = 3, and Sig. = .08.

proactive governance. Private ownership is associated with power focused on a relatively few officials, decentralized power, and a stress by the board on the external linkage functions. Conversely, public ownership is associated with large numbers of officials being involved in governance, centralization of power, and stress on internal administration.

The element within ownership most responsible for these relationships is the leverage afforded by appropriations. The strongest linkages between context and structure are associated with appropriations. Hospitals receiving an appropriation tend to have an "older" board (not to have switched from trustee to hospital board control), to have a relatively large number of officials and groups involved in governance, to be internally oriented, passive, and perceived as ineffectual. The absence of appropriations tends to produce the opposite results.

POLICY IMPLICATIONS

Of the four contextual variables, three have significant policy implications. The first is the implication of the market and political environment. University-owned hospitals have clearly entered an era in which they will be constrained by both greater market competition and regulatory controls of state government. Hospitals in group I in our study will experience much greater constraint than those in groups II and III. If the previous experience of those in group I is applicable to groups II and III as the latter enter this era, it would suggest that governing boards of the latter university hospitals become less concerned with internal administration and more concerned with linking the university hospital to its external environment.

Secondly, the boards of hospitals in groups II and III should become more proactive in the exercise of their governance functions. This means in the case of publicly owned university hospitals that officials of the state and the university should permit the operational board of the university hospital to change its function from management to governance, and to increase the level of their proactivity. This proactivity may involve looking to the state for support and protection, as will be proposed in chapter 7.

The implications from the ownership and appropriation categories are less clear, partly because of the high degree of redundancy in these two categories. But there is also no way of knowing the relationship between greater competition and regulation. The state could behave in one of several ways—all unpredictable. Perhaps, as competition and regulation increase, states will offset the dysfunctional effects of these two factors through increased appropriations. On the other hand, a state may ease regulations as competition becomes a greater regulatory influence on costs and prices. Or, it may permit competition and regulation to take their full toll—forcing a university hospital to become more efficient.

We cannot predict which of these courses of action will occur. It does seem reasonable to suggest, however, that regardless of which conditions actually exist in the market and regulatory environments, hospitals will need governing bodies that place their interests first and that have flexibility in governance decisions. In this regard, the private university hospitals in the past are a model for public university hospitals in the future. According to this logic, public university hospitals and those receiving the higher appropriations need governing bodies that are constituted expressly for the purpose of governing the hospital, that function more to link it to its environment than to handle internal administration, that are proactive in the exercise of responsibilities, and that concentrate on governance rather than management. Of course, the difficulty for the public university hospital will be to gain this measure of independence without losing its appropriation!

REFERENCES

1. Kelly, N.L. A four-cell typology to hospital teaching status. *Inquiry* 21(1984):276–86.
2. Butler, P.W., J.D. Bentley, and R.M. Knapp. Today's teaching hospitals: Old stereotypes and new realities. *Annals of Internal Medicine* 93(October 1980):4.
3. Crispell, K.R., et al. *The organization and governance of academic health centers: Presentation of findings. Vol. 2.* Washington, D.C.: Association of Academic Health Centers, 1980.
4. Elazar, D.J. *American federalism: A view from the states.* New York: Thomas Y. Crowell Co., 1966, pp. 84–126.
5. Sharkansky, I. The utility of Elazar's political culture. *Policy* 2(1969): 66–83.
6. Lammers, W.W. Personal correspondence dated September 27, 1982.
7. Morehouse, S.M. *State politics, parties and policy.* New York: Holt, Rinehart & Winston, 1981, pp. 500–501, 513–14.
8. Grumm, J.G. The effects of legislative structure on legislative performance. In *State and urban politics: Readings in comparative public policy,* edited by R.I. Hofferbert and I. Sharkansky. Boston: Little, Brown & Co., 1971, pp. 299–322.
9. Gray, V. Innovation in the states: A diffusion study. *American Political Science Review* 67(1973):1174–85.

10. Grumm, Legislative structure.
11. Pfeffer, J. Size, composition, and function of hospital boards of directors: A study of organization-environment linkage. *Administrative Science Quarterly* 18(1973):349–64.
12. Zald, M.N. The power and functions of boards of directors: A theoretical synthesis. *American Journal of Sociology* 75(1969):97–111.
13. Pfeffer, J. Size and composition of corporate boards of directors: The organization and its environment. *Administrative Science Quarterly* 17(1972):218–28.
14. Elling, R.H., and S. Halebsky. Organizational differentiation and support: A conceptual framework. *Administrative Science Quarterly* 6(1961): 185–209.
15. Pfeffer, Hospital boards.
16. Price, J.L. The impact of governing boards on organizational effectiveness and morale. *Administrative Science Quarterly* 8(1963):361–78.
17. Mace, M.L. The president and the board of directors. *Harvard Business Review* 50(March–April 1972):37–49.
18. Marris, R., and A. Wood. *The corporate economy: Growth, competition and innovative potential.* Cambridge, Mass.: Harvard University Press, 1971, pp. 1–15.
19. Soman, P., and T. Freidman. *Life and death on the corporate battlefield: How companies win, lose, survive.* New York: Simon and Schuster, 1982, chap. 4.
20. Unterman, I., and R.H. Davis. The strategy gap in not-for-profits. *Harvard Business Review* 60(May–June 1982):30–34.
21. Kovner, A.R. Hospital board members as policy-makers: Role, priorities, and qualifications. *Medical Care* 12(1974):971–82.
22. Terrill, R.C. Governance of university hospitals. Ann Arbor, Mich.: University Microfilms International (Ph.D. Dissertation, University of Indiana, 1978).

FOUR

Measuring University Hospital Performance

In chapter 3 we examined the contextual and governance variables that form one view of the university hospital's environment. In this chapter we focus on a concept closely associated with governance—performance. The new variables introduced here will give us a different perspective on the university hospital's environment, and allow us in a later chapter (chapter 6) to establish a still more comprehensive view.

"Performance" has many meanings in the university hospital context. A university hospital can perform well in providing a site for education, or for research, or for patient care. It can perform well in the sense of doing these with high quality, or doing them with high efficiency (low cost). Some university hospitals may be expected to show a comfortable surplus; others—because of their nonprofit status—may be expected to break even, and to have a large loss or large surplus and would be equally indicative of poor performance or at least poor projection. Most important, different groups influential in the hospital may define "good performance" very differently.

The problem here is made more difficult because the many facets of this concept are difficult to define precisely, and costly to measure accurately. The quality of medical care is the most obvious example, but defining and measuring the quality of support for education and research is equally difficult. An operational definition of efficiency is also difficult, and indeed there is at present no satisfactory method for separating educational costs from those of patient care so that a cost per unit of care can be defined. And what is a unit of care? Even at this fundamental level of definition there is no commonly accepted measure of output.

The problem with defining performance is further aggravated by a changing set of expectations and values. For example, we may argue that quality of care is a measure of performance. But in this era of cost containment, quality of care is important so long as it is delivered at reasonable cost. In other words, quality at any cost is not acceptable to insurers, to payers, and increasingly to the medical professional as well. Moreover, the criteria used to define performance are unstable. This instability stems from the changing expectations of those who have influence over the hospital—its constituencies—all of whom define its performance differently. It is difficult for hospitals to anticipate their constituencies' changing expectations quickly enough to do anything about them.

The perspective of population ecology, which considers whether or not an organization survives, is particularly applicable here: if an organization cannot deviate from its established routines, the changing environment will catch it unaware. But using "survive/not survive" as a performance criterion is not practical or relevant to policy. First of all, no university hospital has failed to survive up to this point. Secondly, to predict nonsurvival actually begs the question. The important or policy-relevant task is to identify the factors and process that enhance survivability.

Defining appropriate measures for university hospital performance is complicated by the question of ownership. The most immediate owner is the parent university, but the actual owner, particularly for university hospitals, is the state. The university expects academic performance from the hospital while the state expects service diversity and excellence.

To reiterate, diverse performance criteria are heaped upon the university hospital; most of it is difficult to quantify. But as hospitals firmly enter the era of competition, there is a growing expectation that the university hospital, too, with all of its attendant missions, has to be able to attain financial solvency. This usually means being able to compete better and be more efficient. For these reasons, even though the demands on university hospitals are legion and performance criteria are divergent, there is sufficient generalized expectation of the hospital from many constituencies to justify using two measures as universally acceptable criteria for university hospital performance: efficiency and viability (financial solvency). More will be said of these two measures later in this chapter. It would be a mistake to assume that efficiency and viability are all that is necessary to gauge university hospital performance, but they are arguably (at least currently) the most common denominators across all hospitals.

The emphasis on efficiency and solvency reflects a changing expectation of public hospitals to perform more like private or commercial hospitals. This may pose a threat to the traditional character of the university hospital and force some of these hospitals to take additional steps to become more competitive, or perhaps more commercial. This is a dilemma that hospital governance and management face: should the hospital respond to competitive pressure or seek state subsidization? Either choice has its inherent risks. Later chapters will show how some states are more amenable to hospital sponsorship than others.

The nature of the state environment has clear consequences for the hospital, including the criteria for performance. Incomplete as efficiency and viability are as criteria for university hospital performance, our judgment is that they are of sufficient universal importance relative to other criteria to justify their use.

The concept of performance adopted in the study is very different from the concept of managerial effectiveness, which is a much narrower construct. Performance is viewed as the goodness of defined hospital outcomes, and it is therefore to be expected that the leadership qualities of the hospital director or the depth of skills in the hospital administrative team will be only part of a larger set of influences on hospital performance. Other influences are the quality of the medical school, the system of controls exercised by the university and the state, the competitive nature of the hospital's environment, and the availability of capital.

UNIVERSITY HOSPITAL PERFORMANCE: A FRAMEWORK

Much of the difficulty related to the measurement of university hospital performance specifically parallels the problems related to the measurement of organizational performance in general. Cameron has developed a useful framework for assessing organizational performance [1]. Emphasizing that there is no best way to judge effectiveness for all organizations, he describes four major perspectives in use today and critiques their strengths and weaknesses:

— Organizational goals perspective
— System-resource perspective

— Internal process perspective
— Strategic constituencies perspective

The most widely used approach emphasizes organizational goals. The closer the organization outputs come to meeting its goals, the more effective the organization. The second, system-resource approach emphasizes the organization's ability to acquire needed resources from the external environment. In contrast to the goals perspective, attention here is on organizational input instead of output.

A third perspective emphasizes the quality of the human organization. The focus of this process approach is on the internal operations or processes in an organization. A highly effective organization is characterized by smooth internal functioning, a stimulating interpersonal atmosphere, and the free flow of information both vertically and horizontally. The fourth perspective, the strategic constituencies or participant-satisfaction perspective, views effectiveness as the extent to which each of the organization's significant constituencies is satisfied with the organization's performance. These constituencies include groups that provide resources for the organization such as suppliers and donors, consumers of the organization's products, employee groups, and groups that regulate the organization's activities, such as government agencies.

Each of these perspectives has its shortcomings. The goals perspective can be flawed because organizations or whole industries may set goals so low that they always achieve them while operating inefficiently. A more serious problem is that persons responsible for goal setting may be unable to agree on goals. In the university hospital context, such conflict arises if the hospital administration believes deeply that net revenues must be positive for the organization to be effective, and the university board of trustees believes just as deeply that a state institution should not profit from the ills of its community. Or, one contingent of the hospital's goal setters may want to emphasize community service, another research and tertiary care. Simply stated, the goals model is unsatisfactory if goals cannot be agreed on or made operational.

The system-resource perspective ignores what an organization does with resources once it secures them. An organization may be successful in securing resources such as money and volunteers from groups in its external environment, but then may waste them or use them inefficiently. Another organization might be less successful in obtaining resources, but use what it does get more efficiently. For example, calling multihospital systems more effective because they can more readily secure capital is a system-resource perspective, but it leaves unanswered the question of how effectively the capital is used. In addition, an organization that is highly successful in obtaining resources can lose the ability to adapt to changes in its resource supply. University medical centers that have had two decades of success in securing federal grants may be ill-fitted to compete in the very different environment of the 1980s [2]. Effectiveness in the long run might differ significantly from effectiveness in the short run because of the loss of adaptability.

The internal process perspective on effectiveness also has weaknesses. An organization might run smoothly yet not achieve its goals; another might be full of internal strife and still be effective. Cameron illustrates this latter possibility with examples from strife-ridden (but winning) baseball teams; those more familar with the academic setting will recognize that the most serene and peaceful medical schools are not always the most productive.

The strategic constituencies perspective is in at least one sense unassailable, for if an organization pleases those constituencies that are truly strategic, it need fear no evil from its environment. But it is also tautological, for in a sense it says no more than "those who succeed, succeed." The difficulties are in knowing which constituencies are strategic, and how to determine if they are pleased.

Clearly most of the criticisms of any one approach assume the perspective of some other approach, and choosing among them must depend on the characteristics of the organization, even more on the purpose the assessment is to serve. This is particularly crucial for organizations such as academic medical centers, which are among groups of organizations often referred to as "organized anarchies" [3]. These organizations are characterized by large and fairly autonomous subunits loosely linked together, and by multiple and ill-defined goals. This fuzziness of goals and internal structure makes organized anarchies particularly difficult to evaluate. Cameron contends that because of the complex nature of organized anarchies, none of the evaluation methods discussed thus far can be used in its pure form. He suggests that an evaluator should consciously restrict analysis to a few key aspects of the organization, and then use the results of a more detailed analysis of those aspects as a proxy measure for organizational effectiveness as a whole.

Cameron proposes several key questions to guide the evaluator of organizational performance, including selection of the critical domain of activity, the key constituencies whose perspectives must be considered, the level of analysis (individual, subunit, organization), and whether short- or long-term effectiveness is of primary interest. He also notes significant issues in the selection of objective and subjective data, and finally the selection of a yardstick (whether comparison is with an ideal standard, with past performance, or with similar organizations).

APPLICATION OF THE FRAMEWORK TO UNIVERSITY HOSPITALS

We have found the questions that Cameron raises useful in developing our own measures. With regard to using objective data or subjective assessments as the basis for performance measures, we have taken the easy (and really the only available) alternative in deciding to depend heavily on the financial and operating data that the cooperating hospitals have authorized us to use. These data come primarily from material submitted annually to the Council on Teaching Hospitals (COTH). The general comparability of data between hospitals from this source is an advantage, for our major interest is in understanding how differences among university hospitals and their environments influence performance. For this reason interhospital comparisons are essential, although the notion of an ideal standard is implicit in several measures (for example, the viability measure).

While one may find it convenient and in many respects accurate to describe university hospitals as organized anarchies, it is also true that such a characterization is not helpful in defining assessment criteria [4]. In spite of its tautological quality the strategic constituencies approach represents the best fit with our study's purpose. Unfortunately there are many constituencies, as our earlier description of the ownership environment made clear. Moreover, the degree to which constituencies are strategic is not uniform from one hospital to the next, although the same ones (state, university administration, medical school and chiefs) within the ownership environment tend to appear. By translating the question from "How satisfied are constituencies?" to "What do they want?" it is possible to identify variables that are more consistent with a goals approach, and to think in terms of that familiar trilogy: teaching, research, and patient care.

This does not resolve the question, for the university hospital's contribution to teaching and research is qualitatively different from its production of patient care, and a measure of hospital performance in these first two areas should not use data that are in fact more descriptive of medical school performance. This is the question of levels and it is a real one, for certain measures of performance may in fact reflect performance of the medical center (of which the university hospital is a subunit) or of the hospital's medical staff (a subunit of the hospital). It is pointless to detail our hopes and disappointments in this area; we were able to index facilities available for education and research through the number of services a hospital offered, and to index the patients available for teaching and research by the number of patients per house officer. While we would have liked to add financial support to facility and patient support, we found no data source of sufficient reliability to do so.

As we mentioned in the beginning of this chapter, for many university hospitals a major interest of their strategic constituencies is the hospital's viability; in the current period of procompetition, this seems to depend more heavily on economic definitions than on any others. We used revenue surplus to index the organization's viability. While this measure reflects performance in the patient care area, it certainly does not index all of its dimensions, most notably the quality of that care. We do not have a measure of quality useful for distinguishing within the rather narrow band of quality differences that exist among university hospitals, and our analysis is necessarily limited by that fact.

A measure of increasing interest is a hospital's efficiency in its use of resources. Concern for efficiency will continue to grow as viability becomes more problematic. Therefore we thought it useful to include an index that seeks to measure resource efficiency. A major exclusion from this index is data on personnel per occupied bed, cost per day, or cost per admission. The reason for this omission is simple. These data also reflect the type of care offered and are thus a positive measure of intensity of services, as well as a negative measure of efficiency. Where possible we sought to exclude measures with such widely divergent and therefore uncertain meanings.

We summarize below the actual content of our performance indices after noting one further weakness. Most data are drawn from the hospitals' fiscal years ending in 1981, although some indices make use of 1979 and 1980 data. At the time of data collection (1982), even the 1981 data were unavailable, and were among the last data received. The use of two-year-old data weakens our conclusions, but the alternatives were less satisfactory and we believe the major conclusions would not be radically altered by having more recent data. Unless otherwise noted, all performance data come from cooperating hospitals' responses to the COTH annual survey [5].

Key Performance Variables

The key performance variables presented here are viability, efficiency, facilities, and the number of patients per house officer.

Viability

Hospital viability is measured in two ways. The first is composed of 1980–81 net revenues less state, county, and city appropriations, expressed as a proportion of 1980–81 total operating expenses (see table 4.1). For example an index value of 0.050 indicates that hospital operating revenues (excluding appropriations) exceeded operating expenses by an average of 5 percent over the two-year period. The second measure includes these appropriations as a part of net revenues (see table 4.2). The financial viability measures thus indicate the degree to which net operating revenues in either case exceeded or fell short of total operating expenses. The first viability index is the ratio of total operating revenues (less appropriations) to total operating expenses. This measure combines data from the fiscal years ending 1980 and 1981.

The strength of the first measure is its universal recognition as the key test of continued viability for organizations that must generate their own revenues. By eliminating appropriations from patient revenues, we eliminate the ambiguities produced by the varying reasons for state appropriations. However, the primary weakness of this measure is that some state appropriations are specifically given to cover indigent care, and are therefore properly treated as patient revenue. It is impos-

Table 4.1 Viability without State Appropriations

	All UHs	Public UHs	Private UHs
Minimum	−0.477		
Maximum	0.078		
Mean	−0.106	−0.157	−0.009
Standard deviation	0.129	0.122	0.077
Hospitals included	49	32	17

Table 4.2 Viability with Appropriations

	All UHs	Public UHs	Private UHs
Minimum	−0.480		
Maximum	0.210		
Mean	0.023	0.018	−0.013
Standard deviation	0.125	0.147	0.162
Hospitals included	47	31	16

sible, not just difficult, to determine what portion of appropriation to each hospital is truly patient revenue. One may also argue that a dollar from appropriations is as good as any other dollar, and a hospital's success in securing such dollars should be taken into account. For this reason, we have included appropriations in the second measure.

Efficiency

The efficiency index is a measure of how efficiently facilities (occupancy), operating capital (receivables), and materials (inventory) are used. Of all the indexes it is probably the one that can be most directly influenced by managerial action. Our efficiency index uses 1981 data for (1) inventory per occupied bed, (2) days revenues in receivables, and (3) occupancy, adjusted for whether the occupancy level is an increase or decrease from the prior year. By not including a measure of personnel utilization, the efficiency measure is less likely to be distorted by large differences in the intensity of case mix.

The first two components were reverse scored so that a higher efficiency score would result from lower inventory, lower days in receivables, and higher occupancy. Each index component was standardized, and appropriate weights were derived from a factor analysis. Cronbach's alpha was calculated and yielded a moderate 0.51. We then factor analyzed the data to make sure that the components rightfully belonged to one index; this resulted in a single-factor solution with 35 percent of the variance explained. This solution indicates that the three components share sufficient common variance to be treated as a single index, thus providing confidence in the reliability of the scale.

A weakness of the index is its partial and incomplete reflection of the multiple components of resource efficiency. Also, because of the standardizing of scores, a hospital's index value has no meaning by itself.

Table 4.3 Efficiency

	All UHs	Public UHs	Private UHs
Minimum	−2.14		
Maximum	1.43		
Mean	0.00	−0.303	0.572
Standard deviation	0.8368	0.7792	0.6268
Hospitals included	52	34	18

Facilities

This index is the number of facilities in the hospital, as defined in the American Hospital Association's annual survey. The AHA defined 53 facilities or services at the time of the study, including such services as intensive care, burn care, hemodialysis, occupational therapy, home care, and CT (computerized tomography) scanner. A hospital with a relatively high number of facilities offers broader teaching and research opportunities by allowing a more complex mix of patients to be served.

The index value for a single hospital is a simple count of the facilities in place.

Although this measure is occasionally used as a structural measure of quality, its use here is primarily to reflect the hospital's ability to provide broad support for the varied teaching, research, and tertiary care interests of the medical staff.

Patients per House Officer

This index uses adjusted patient days (from the efficiency index) in the numerator and the number of house officers as the denominator to specify the number of patients per house officer.

The data used to compute this index come from two sources. The number of house staff at each hospital was taken from the 1982 COTH Directory of Educational Programs and Services. Other data were taken from the hospitals' annual survey responses to COTH for the fiscal year ending in 1981.

This index indicates how many patients each house officer might oversee during an average day. A higher number of patients per house officer is presumed to lead to a higher quality learning experience for the house staff, because they then have exposure to more cases. At some point the number of patients could become too large; however, in the hospitals under study, the largest number was 5.6—a number we believe is below that danger point.

RELATIONSHIPS AMONG PERFORMANCE INDEXES

Relationships among the four performance indexes provide useful information. Those that are grossly inconsistent with existing knowledge about university hospitals raise questions about the validity of the indexes, and therefore relations among them need to be reviewed first from a critical perspective. This activity occupied much of our time, and has led to substantial revisions in our performance measures. Sec-

Table 4.4 Hospital Facilities

	All UHs	Public UHs	Private UHs
Minimum	24.0		
Maximum	47.0		
Mean	38.3	38.6	37.7
Standard deviation	4.39	4.14	4.87
Hospitals included	51	33	18

Table 4.5 Patients Per House Officer

	All UHs	Public UHs	Private UHs
Minimum	1.19		
Maximum	5.55		
Mean	2.40	2.29	2.62
Standard deviation	0.8463	0.8348	0.8538
Hospitals included	48	32	16

ondly, relationships among the indexes illuminate certain characteristics of the university hospitals and represent in this way an insight into the nature of those hospitals.

Table 4.6 shows correlation matrixes for relations among the performance variables. It includes a separate matrix of correlations for all university hospitals, for public university hospitals, and for private university hospitals.

Efficiency and viability are strongly correlated both in the full set and in public hospitals, but weakly correlated in private hospitals. The weaker relation among the private hospitals is surprising, and contrary to our expectation.

The number of facilities has a negative and generally weak relation to the patients-per-house-officer measure, suggesting that these two indexes of support for teaching and research operate quite independently of each other. An exception to this is in the private hospitals, where the patients-per-house-officer index has a strong negative correlation with facilities. Possibly hospitals with a strong research emphasis have more residents, and have them longer, while those that badly need to avoid deficits may economize both on house officers and facilities. It may be that these tendencies are most pronounced among

Table 4.6 Correlations among Performance Indicators

PPHO	−.2245		
EFF	.0928	.3243*	
VIAB	−.2492	.2802	.5333†
	FAC	PPHO	EFF

Set 1
All cases—outlier removed
52 hospitals

PPHO	−.0686		
EFF	.2173	.2208	
VIAB	−.2308	.1860	.4320‡
	FAC	PPHO	EFF

Set 2
All public hospitals—outliers removed
34 hospitals

PPHO	−.5963‡		
EFF	.0811	.3955	
VIAB	−.2494	.2566	.1239
	FAC	PPHO	EFF

Set 3
All private hospitals—outliers removed
18 hospitals

Note: outliers defined as in excess of 4 s.d.s. from the mean.
*Significant at the .01 level.
†Significant at the .001 level.
‡Significant at the .05 level.

the private hospitals. Facilities have a uniformly negative relation to viability and patients-per-house-officer a uniformly positive relation, though both are weak.

Efficiency is uncorrelated with facilities, suggesting that hospitals with many or few services are able to score well on efficient use of resources. This observation was abundantly supported in our field studies, and is related to findings elsewhere. Scott and Shortell, reviewing studies of hospital performance that relate cost performance to quality of care, suggest that efficiency and quality may be positively correlated [6]. The relationships observed were not strong, however, and the most that can confidently be said is that efficiency and good quality care need not be mutually exclusive. The implication of the studies is that at least some managerial actions or environmental conditions can improve both factors simultaneously.

Perhaps the central observation we can make about the performance indexes is that they show a significant independence from each other, suggesting that we are tapping truly separate dimensions of performance. Evidently there are multiple dimensions on which the performance of university hospitals may be judged; the diverse data used to form these performance indexes, together with the substantial independence shown in the intercorrelations, offer some hope that we have avoided a unidimensional definition of performance.

SUMMARY

The approach to performance adopted in this study acknowledges the presence of strategic constituencies that make demands on the university hospital. The central importance of these constituencies varies among university hospitals; therefore, it is not possible to select one or two measures of performance as equally relevant to all. The different dimensions of performance need not, and do not, move together. Increasingly, the question of survival of the university hospital has caused the various constituencies to give more weight to the viability of the hospital, and in this study measures have been selected to give more weight to that performance criterion.

The viability measures selected are partial and incomplete indexes of performance for three reasons: the concept to be measured is often difficult to make operational; definitions of goodness vary from hospital to hospital because of differing objectives; data are often unavailable, or available only after a substantial time lag.

The general concept of performance we have adopted is not an evaluative one. A hospital that has few facilities is not judged to be poor, while one with many is judged good. Although service to education and research, efficiency, and surplus are selected because some constituency wants them to be high, the index value achieved is expected to be a product of multiple causes, including some outside the control of any constituency or coalition among them. Therefore, in an evaluative sense, a hospital with a deficit may be making better use of resources than one with a surplus. Likewise, a hospital with a lower efficiency may be adapting to a hostile environment with great skill, while one with higher efficiency may be doing little to take advantage of its (possibly far more supportive) environment.

The central value of these performance measures is the description they provide of how well the university hospitals are doing, without any attribution of reasons. The effort to find reasons is the goal of the following chapters.

REFERENCES

1. Cameron, K. Critical questions in assessing organizational effectiveness. *Organization Dynamics* 9(Autumn 1980):66–80.
2. Ebert, R., and S. Brown. Academic health centers. *New England Journal of Medicine* 308(1983):1200–1208.
3. Cameron, Organizational effectiveness.
4. Lutz, F. W. Tightening up loose couplings in organizations of higher education. *Administrative Science Quarterly* 27(1982):653–69.
5. Isaacs, J. *COTH survey of university-owned teaching hospitals' financial and general operating data. 1979, 1980, 1981*. Washington, D.C.: Department of Teaching Hospitals, Association of American Medical Colleges, 1981, 1982, 1983.
6. Scott, W.R., and S. Shortell. Organizational performance: Managing for efficiency and effectiveness. In *Health care management* edited by S. Shortell and A. Kaluzny. New York: John Wiley, 1983.

FIVE

Structure of the Political Environment

In chapter 3 we demonstrated how the governance of hospitals is strongly related to the political environment—for example, the amount of state appropriations and subsequent state influence on the university hospital board, the number of university administrators involved with decision making, and so on. Now, we take the question of environment a step further. Does a variation among states in business or political climate—that is, its culture—determine, affect, or predict the way university hospitals are governed? In this chapter we explain the term "political environment" to include ways of doing things. In particular we examine the differences in the relationships between public and private university hospitals and their state culture, and the resulting governance situations.

HISTORICAL BACKGROUND—THE UNIVERSITY HOSPITAL AND THE STATE

Historically, university hospitals were funded (and governed) entirely by the university and its medical school. Gradually, however, the state and other sources increased their funding, so that by the late 1960s over 40 percent of hospital revenues were provided by public sources, compared with 20 percent or less from the university. As a result, the hospitals became more dependent on the outside environment.

Unfortunately, this outside environment has recently become unpredictable and even hostile. A major factor is the federal government, which has changed the method of payment for health care. Its formerly generous cost-based reimbursement approach has become a fixed-fee approach that penalizes high-cost, inefficient hospitals—which university hospitals often are, because of their educational mission. Moreover the federal government has also encouraged competition as the preferred method of regulating hospitals; as a result, state governments have stepped in to fill the regulatory void [1]. A third factor is the trend toward HMOs and other multiinstitutional integration within the industry. This poses a serious threat to sources of patient referrals to university hospitals, because many university hospitals are unable to join similar groups. The unfortunate fact is that university hospitals no longer face a simple choice between university, marketplace, or state regulatory controls; they are constrained by all three.

In previous research and in the field study phase of the current research, we observed that private university-owned hospitals enjoyed greater autonomy than state university-owned hospitals. Secondly, we saw considerable variation in the autonomy enjoyed by the various state university-owned hospitals. In general, it seemed that southern state governments seemed more pro-business or laissez faire toward business in the private sector than northern state governments, and that southern states imposed considerably more bureaucratic constraints on their universities and university hospitals than did northern states. In many southern states, the state and the parent university often seemed to their university hospital to be more a part of the regulatory environment than a part of ownership. That is, some hospitals seemed to face "two environments," the same market and regulatory environment faced by all business and the additional constraints imposed by a highly-constraining, not always supportive state government [2].

There appeared to be a political environment that varied dramatically between the states and had direct and significant effects on the operations of state government at all levels—extending down to state universities and their hospitals. Industry has long been keenly aware of a phenomenon known as the 'business climate index' that measures a variety of variables bearing on the profitability of for-profit enterprises [3]. A state with a high or favorable business climate index would have low wages, low employment and workers' compensation rates, fewer unionized workers, etc. With a single number, therefore, businesses thinking of relocating to more favorable environs can know which states are more favorable. The so-called 'southern strategy', by which basic industries in the snow belt have relocated to the sun belt, is thus explained by this index rather than the weather. The recent publicity surrounding the siting of the Saturn division of GM in Tennessee highlighted the factors making that state's business climate favorable for automotive production.

In like manner, we wondered if there were an index of the political climate in each state that could explain systematic and observable differences in the laws and governmental operations of the states as they relate to the operation of state universities and their hospitals. It turned out that there is a well-researched phenomenon in political science known as "political culture" that measures the political realm as effectively as the business climate index does the economic sector [4]. Our research, therefore, relates measures of political culture and the market to hospital governance and performance. University-owned hospitals face increased constraints from regulations, market competition, and bureaucratic controls of states and universities, and we tested whether the character of these constraints was reliably summarized and predictable by reference to measures of the political climate of the states.

THEORETICAL PERSPECTIVE

How one views the environment depends on where one is standing—in other words, what the unit of analysis is. We have specified the university hospital as the unit of analysis; this makes its university, and the state's politics and economy, simply two parts of the university hospital's task environment. According to Churchman, the environment of such a focal social system (e.g., the university hospital) includes those elements that are relevant to but not controllable by that focal system [5]. For a university hospital, the relevant environment is the whole state, based on goals and patient referral patterns.

Astley and Van de Ven have developed a useful metatheory that categorizes theories in terms of two dimensions: level of analysis (micro or macro) and assumptions about control (whether environment controls the organization, or the other way around)[6]. Within this framework our research into university hospitals would support the salience of the external influence perspective, that is, the university hospital is the dependent variable acted upon by the environment. Such external influence is felt both at the micro level of analysis (the individual university hospital) and the macro level (the entire universe of university hospitals). According to this perspective the organization's structure functions to meet given goals of the larger social system—in this case, the state.

In our study we viewed "political culture" as an independent variable exogenous to the model. As one might expect, political scientists do not agree about how to define this term. We have used the definition most relevant to our organizational-science model and to the policies we hope to affect by our study: political culture is "the dominant traditions about what constitutes proper government action" [7,8,9]. There are two major traditions, or subcultures, that comprise radically different ways of viewing government's role in society; these subcultures are called "market" and "commonwealth." Somewhere in between the two is a third type that can be called "elitist" or "traditional." These three subcultures actually range along a continuum, but for a clear initial understanding of them it is easiest to think of them as separate types, as shown in table 5.1.

It is important to remember that every state contains elements of all three subcultures, but it is possible for one of them to predominate. This three-subculture perspective, first proposed and tested by Elazar and Sharkansky, has been replicated by Johnson, who showed it to be independent of economic conditions and strongly related to the religious affiliation of the population [10,11,12].

In the pure individualist or market perspective, public relationships are products of bargaining among individuals and groups, who act out of self-interest to exercise power and bring about a just society. In contrast, in the moralist or "commonwealth" perspective the whole people share certain moral principles and an undivided interest in the state as a vehicle that will bring about a just society. The elitist or "traditionalist" perspective reflects an older, precommercial royalist attitude, in which a hierarchical society expects and authorizes those at the top of the social ladder to dominate in government. According to this perspective, government may properly initiate action if it serves to perpetuate the ruling elite and the existing status quo of the social order.

As table 5.1 indicates, the three types view government bureaucracy and the need for welfare legislation quite differently. Clearly, the state's role is much stronger in the moralistic society, spending more on welfare and consequently exerting greater control over these areas with more welfare legislation, workers' compensation, and so on. It is not surprising, then, that the moralistic subcultures tend to score lowest on the business climate index.

In sum, political science provides a model similar to that of the microdeterministic perspective within organization science. Political subcultures within the various states, together with economic or mar-

Table 5.1 Characteristics of Three Political Subcultures

Factor	Moralist (Commonwealth)	Elitist (Traditionalist)	Individualist (Market)
Human motivation	Shared moral principles	Perpetuate status quo	Self-interest
View of government bureaucracy	Carries out people's common wishes	Should exist only to perpetuate status quo; instrument of control by elite	Ambivalent
Attitude toward welfare laws	Initiated by state; more laws, more spending	Only when forced	Only when forced

ket factors, are a part of the task environment of all university hospitals, especially those owned by state universities. These subcultures are relevant to three topics important to this study, public welfare, education, and centralization of decision making.

RESEARCH QUESTIONS

We asked two questions in this part of the study:

1. How well does the political-culture variable relate to and summarize key characteristics of the political system and policy outcomes of the states in which university hospitals are located?
2. What are the effects of ownership on the university or, subsequently, on university hospital governance and performance?

The first question grew out of our primary thesis that the political environments of the states are heterogenous. That is, there is no single institutional environment that fully captures the variation in political and economic factors comprising the task environments of the various university hospitals. So, for policy and theoretical purposes, it is important to characterize the variety within the political and economic environments constraining university hospitals.

The second question grew out of our second thesis, that university hospital owners (such as university officers and state government officials) can sometimes act in the posture of outsiders toward their university hospital, constraining and inhibiting its best interests rather than supporting them. From a business perspective, such owner behavior would be similar to that of corporate management acting contrary to the best interests of the stockholders (the real owners). In either case, management views the owners more as part of the environment to contend with than a part of the organization.

We hypothesized that a state-owned university hospital receiving a state appropriation would be more affected by the political environment than a private university hospital receiving the same appropriation. By the same token, a university with larger state appropriations would be more dependent on the state than one receiving a large share of its revenues from research grants and contracts. In sum, both ownership (whether private or public) and appropriations (dependence on state and university subsidies) would have a profound influence on governance.

The connection of welfare to university hospitals is clear and strong: it provides charity care and Medicaid-paid care. In moralistic states, poor people are more likely to get care in hospitals other than the state's own university hospital, and if they are treated in a university hospital, they are more likely to be covered by Medicaid.

The attitude toward higher education (thus, funding and control of universities and other hospitals) is complex. Paradoxically a moralistic society, despite its tendency toward bureaucratic controls, is more likely to permit a university greater autonomy.

The concept of autonomy is worth discussing in some detail. Autonomy is much more likely when a university is owned or controlled by a constitutionally authorized university board that is not subject to close control by the political system. Such boards are more likely in moralistic subcultures [13]. Secondly, there seems to be some association between the university's independence or administrative distance from the state and the ability of the university to generate its own sources of revenues through philanthropy and research. Apparently more autonomous university administrators are inclined to seek sources of support independent of the state, and private citizens are more inclined to give to universities they see as less tied to political control. (One could understand a citizen being reluctant to donate large sums to a public university already receiving virtually all its revenues from tax-supported sources.) Hence university autonomy, possibly originating within a moralistic subculture, eventually culminates in greater financial independence through endowment and research funding [14].

METHODS

We obtained data describing the independent variables—the political and market environments surrounding university hospitals—from sources independent of university hospitals. Market data were obtained from U.S. government census reports, the American Medical Association, and the Conference of State Manufacturers' Associations. Measures of the political system and political system policy outcomes were obtained from sources within the political science literature and U.S. census reports. Measures of university finances were initially collected by the National Center for Education Statistics and subsequently analyzed by the National Center for Higher Education Management Systems. Measures of hospital performance were obtained by permission from the Association of American Medical Colleges' Council of Teaching Hospitals and from the American Medical Association.

In chapter 3, we correlated 4 contextual variables with 7 governance variables (size of the university hospital board, etc.). Here we examine the relationship between subculture types and 14 environment variables for each of the 33 states having university hospitals, as shown in table 5.2. (Note that 13 of these variables were also used in chapter 3; only the "business climate index" is new here.)

Since the difference between moralistic and individualistic is essentially a continuum, we have presented the results of each of the 14 correlations as they relate to one end of the continuum: moralistic. Thus, a strong correlation between a variable and political culture means that the variable is correlated with characteristics of a moralistic society. The null hypothesis—that there is no correspondence between political culture and the hospital's political and economic environment at the state level—was tested with a two-tailed test and rejected at the $p = .05$ level for 10 of the 14 variables.

FINDINGS

Political Culture

As might be expected, political culture is significantly related to four of the five political system variables. In a moralistic political culture, legislatures tend to be innovative and to be judged effective. This tends to follow from their high interparty competition and wealth. Although the relationship was not statistically significant, there is also a tendency for their governors to be "strong" (as measured by their power to make appointments). Moralistic states tend to subsidize disproportionately the federal government by paying out more federal taxes than the federal government returns to the state.

Of the four policy outputs variables (6 through 9), two have a statistically significant relationship to political culture. Moralistic po-

Table 5.2 Institutional Environment Correlates of the Political Culture of the State ($N = 33$ States)

	r	p
INSTITUTIONAL ENVIRONMENT (9)		
Political System		
1. Federal subsidy to state ($ from federal government: $ to federal government)	−.55	.001
2. Legislative innovation (speed—months—in passing model legislation)	−.80	<.001
3. Legislative effectiveness (rating: high number equals high rating)	.69	<.001
4. Interparty competition (high number equals high competition between political parties)	.83	<.001
5. Governor's appointment powers (high number equals high number of appointments)	.23	N.S.
Policy Outputs		
6. Welfare burden (state & local government $ expenditures adjusted for wealth/personal income of residents)	.61	<.001
7. Redistribution of income to the poor (benefits received by the poor: taxes paid by the poor)	.54	.001
8. Coordination of higher education (high number equals high central coordination by state)	−.26	N.S.
9. State expenditures per FTE student in major universities	−.04	N.S.
MARKET ENVIRONMENT (5)		
10. Personal income per capita, 1979	.74	<.001
11. Population, 1980	.17	N.S.
12. Urbanization (% population in SMSAs, 1975)	.38	.03
13. M.D.s in specialty practice per 100,000 population	.38	.03
14. Business climate index (high number indicates "good" business climate, i.e., low payroll taxes, etc.)	−.40	.02

litical cultures tend to legislate relatively more generous welfare systems that are financed by higher-income groups. That is, their programs are supported by progressive income taxes that redistribute wealth rather than regressive sales taxes that place equally heavy burdens on all income groups.

How well a state supports welfare is a proxy for how well a state makes provision for health and hospital care throughout the state. In effect, the better the welfare system in general, the less burden the state's university hospital(s) must carry. For example, the fact that there are county hospitals in a state means the university hospital is less likely to be the only provider of care for indigents—which has consequences for the image and financial performance of the university hospital. (Indigent care is typically not adequately paid for by states, and the presence of a sizeable proportion of indigents together with the formal designation of "charity hospital" tends to reduce the appeal of a university hospital to paying patients.) Hence, the linkage between a state's general welfare system and the role and performance of its university hospital is direct and important.

Although the relationship is statistically nonsignificant, moralistic states tend to operate their universities in a more decentralized manner ($r = .26$). Their universities tend to be insulated from direct state controls and political involvement by having separate boards mandated by the state's constitution. In contrast, individualistic and traditional states tend toward greater state control, that is, states that favor market controls for the private sector actually favor bureaucratic controls for their own state-run agencies.

Finally, there is no direct relationship between political culture and the level of financial support a state provides its universities. Education is a universal aspect of all political subcultures, being highly valued in all of them, and the share of state budgets devoted to it tends to be equal across the states.

Political culture is significantly related to four of the five "market environment" variables (10 through 13). It is apparent that university hospitals in a moralistic culture have the most benign economic climate. Moralistic states tend to be wealthier (though not more populous), to be more urbanized, and to have a higher proportion of physician specialists. Thus, a university hospital in such a state has more patients who can pay their bills. Moreover, because of the state's better welfare system, the hospital is less likely to have to absorb the costs of those who cannot pay their bills.

Finally, variable 14 shows that a moralistic culture tends to have a poorer business climate as judged by private industry. That is, businesses shoulder higher payroll taxes, pay higher wages, tend more often to be unionized, and are subject to more stringent zoning and planning laws.

What specific, predictable results does this variance in political cultures have for the university hospital? Consider the following phenomena.

Currently, ten states have mandatory rate-setting policies that cover all third-party payers. Seven of these are "moralistic" states [15]. Similarly, a necessary prelude to almost any kind of state rate-review or rate-setting program is uniform accounting or reporting requirements for hospitals, and in 1983 four other states enacted laws establishing some type of hospital reporting system. Three of these four states are moralistic.

Ownership

Our second research question was, "does it make any difference, given a political subculture, whether a university hospital is privately owned or state owned?" The results of the analysis of ownership are presented in table 5.3.

The 11 dependent variables in table 5.3 represent characteristics of successive levels within the ownership or bureaucratic hierarchy: medical school (variable 1), university (variables 2 and 3), state (variables 4 and 5), university hospital governance (variables 6 through 9), and university hospital performance (variables 10 and 11). Because private university hospitals tend to be disproportionately sited in "moralistic" states, we held political culture constant while testing the effects of ownership. Consequently we used covariance analysis with political culture as the covariate. The unit of analysis, the university hospital, was divided by ownership into private university-owned

Table 5.3 Analysis of Covariance

Dependent Variable	Covariate (Political Culture)			Ownership (Public/Private*)			
	Beta	S.E.	p	$\bar{X}$	Adj. $\bar{X}$	d.f.	p
1. Hospital efficiency index (Chapters 2, 4, & 7)	.099	.04	.02				
Public				−.29	−.29	[1,47]	<.001
Private				.62	.62		
2. Percent hospital profits, excluding appropriations (Chapters 2, 4, & 7)	.013	.006	.03				
Public				.88	.88	[1,47]	<.001
Private				1.00	1.00		
3. Governance vs. management emphasis (Chapter 3)	.02	0.05	N.S.				
Public				1.9	1.0	[1,47]	N.S.
Private				2.14	2.14		

Continued

Table 5.3 Continued

Dependent Variable	Covariate (Political Culture)			Ownership (Public/Private*)			
	Beta	S.E.	p	X̄	Adj. X̄	d.f.	p
4. Board's proactivity (Chapter 3)	−.82	0.84	N.S.				
Public				.89	.89	[1,47]	.08
Private				.07	.07		
5. Percent hospital revenue from state appropriations (Chapters 3 & 7)	−1.18	1.24	N.S.				
Public				17.4	17.4	[1,45]	.01
Private				0.07	0.08		
6. Percent charity care by hospital (Chapter 6)	−1.44	0.78	.07				
Public				17.4	17.2	[1,44]	N.S.
Private				14.1	14.8		
7. Medical school rank (Chapter 7)	−4.7	1.72	.009				
Public				55.3	55.0	[1,45]	.045
Private				35.1	35.9		
8. Percent university revenue from appropriations (Chapter 7)	−1.76	0.52	.001				
Public				52.5	52.1	[1,40]	<.001
Private				8.6	10.4		
9. Percent university revenue from grants (Chapter 7)	1.50	0.49	.004				
Public				19.9	20.0	[1,46]	<.001
Private				31.7	31.6		
10. Centralization governance power (Chapter 11)	.12	.006	N.S.				
Public				.38	.38	[1,47]	<.001
Private				.24	.24		
11. Percent dispersion governance power (Chapter 11)	.025	.068	N.S.				
Public				1.57	1.57	[1,47]	.02
Private				0.69	0.69		

Note: Signs defined in terms of correlation with moralistic political culture. The equal-slope assumption was met in all the above tests.
*Public university hospitals coded as zero; private university hospitals coded as 1.

As in the previous analysis, we present our results in terms of correlation with a moralistic political subculture. (The test of the null hypothesis—that there is no correspondence between political culture and ownership on the one hand and characteristics of the university hospital's ownership environment on the other hand—is reported below.)

Political culture is significantly related to 6 of the 11 variables tested, and ownership is significantly related to 9. In general, findings show that political culture is related to the nature of the university and its hospital's performance, whether public or private, but is not related to the hospital's governance. Apparently a university acts as a shield or buffer, preventing the political culture and system from strongly influencing how the university governs its hospital.

The more moralistic the culture, the more beneficial the influence, for two reasons. First, universities in moralistic cultures tend to be less dependent upon state appropriations and more dependent upon funds generated through research. These universities are not only more independent of the state, they are more research oriented. Their medical schools mirror this by being more research oriented—as indicated by their higher rankings. Second, university hospitals in moralistic cultures have to provide less charity care, presumably because the state's welfare system either makes care in the university hospitals less necessary or pays the hospital more adequately for that care through Medicaid. These university hospitals, not being saddled with a primary mission of indigent care, can focus on tertiary-level, superspecialty care consistent with the medical school's research emphasis. This focus on superspecialty care has another advantage: it differentiates their product in the manner most advantageous to them in their highly competitive markets.

Our findings show that there is no relationship between culture and the university hospital's dependence upon the state for appropriations. Similarly, university hospital governance, as measured by our four variables, is unaffected by political culture. That is, lower financial dependence reduces the state's leverage for directly influencing governance. However, even though political culture does not influence governance, it does influence performance; university hospitals in moralistic cultures are both more efficient and profitable. This influence, rather than operating through governance, operates through the very nature of the university, the medical school, and the welfare system.

If we hold political culture constant, ownership has an additional strong influence on universities and their hospitals. Presumably, political culture explains the influence of the nature of state government. By holding political culture constant, therefore, we are examining not the nature of state government as it varies among the states, but the mere fact of state ownership per se as compared with private ownership. The question explored here is how ownership per se affects universities and their hospitals. Our overall observation of the data is that state ownership has deleterious effects upon university hospitals.

As one would expect, state university hospitals depend more upon state appropriations. (This is not tautological; some private university hospitals, primarily those in Pennsylvania, receive modest state appropriations.) Private hospitals depend more upon funds generated through research. This is partly due to autocorrelation (the greater the proportion of total university revenues from appropriations, the less there is from research) and partly from the fact that the unavailability of appropriations to the private hospitals forces them to seek funds from research and philanthropy. This difference in emphasis is mirrored in their medical schools, with those in private universities being more research oriented. As we discussed in chapter 3, state ownership is associated with governing boards that are less proactive, more centralized, and more diffuse. State ownership means that more officials and higher levels of officials are involved in their hospital's governance, and those doing the governing are passive rather than proactive.

Being owned by the state does not, per se, imply that the state university hospital will perform a strong role in providing charity care: private university hospitals provide as much charity care as state hospitals. Charity care is more a function of the general welfare system and is, therefore, independent of the higher education system—consistent with the functional specialization characterizing most state governments.

Finally, state influence is associated with lower efficiency and operating profits in state university hospitals.

The one obvious benefit of state ownership—appropriations—may offset the other dysfunctional effects. If appropriations are added back to our measure of profits (variable 11), the difference between public and private disappears. That is, even though some state hospitals are not financially self-sufficient, the state's subsidy compensates for this operating deficit.

IMPLICATIONS FOR THEORY

The classic Aston studies opened the way to operationalizing the concept of organizational dependence [16]. Their approach involved seven scales and included measures that our research has shown to be useful and important to understanding university hospitals. They distinguished between market and ownership dependence, and public accountability of the parent organization. In our research we have established that for university hospitals, ownership is an influential environmental factor and that public and private owners provide quite different constraints. Our findings are consistent with the Aston studies in regard to the relationship between environmental dependence and structure; that is, publicly owned university hospitals are more dependent through appropriations from their owners, the state, and their governance is more centralized and diffuse.

Our ownership findings also have implications for the population-ecology and protected-organizations perspectives (see chapter 2) regarding the relationship between environment and organizational forms. "Dependence" is a key term here. The more an organization depends on the ownership environment (for example, on state subsidies), the more it is sheltered from the competitive environment, and the more likely it is to have a governance structure conforming to its ownership environment. Governing boards perform two primary functions: internal administration, and linking the hospital with relevant external environments [17]. Private university-owned hospitals must stress linkage with external sources of patient care and philanthropic dollars, and success in this requires greater control at lower levels by hospital and medical school officials. Conversely, state university-owned hospitals must secure public funds and approvals, and doing this requires governance at a higher level within the hierarchy of owners, and involves more participants in the governance process.

According to our findings, therefore, success in competitive markets calls for more streamlined university hospital governance—more decentralized, and with fewer organizational entities involved. Conversely, success in coping with owners is associated with more organizational entities being involved in a more centralized way.

We have also established that the political dimension of environments is relevant to research on university hospitals. Hospitals have too long been considered a single species facing a single, national environment. We have clearly documented here the highly variable nature of state environments, including their political characteristics, and have shown how the internal structures of university hospitals vary accordingly. Therefore it seems reasonable to conclude that we are dealing with multiple organizational forms and environments. On both theoretical and policy grounds it is important to recognize the political dimension of these environments, and to study university hospitals in groupings according to those environments. At minimum, it seems feasible to classify these environments along two dimensions:

ownership (public and private), and political system (market and government regulation).

POLICY IMPLICATIONS

There are two major policy options that have been seriously considered as methods of dealing with cost, quality, and access to health care in the United States: competition, and regulation and rate controls. Since the health system currently faces (and will be facing) a combination of both, the question is how our findings bear on this probable future for university hospitals. Federal and state governments are encouraging both forms of control, but our research indicates that it is the variance of state actions that will have important implications for university hospital viability.

As we have stated, "moralistic" states have both high market competition and strict regulation. If market competition increases further, and if regulation becomes more severe, their university hospitals may find the strain intense. Moralistic states that continue to stress both forms of constraint will provide a much more hostile environment than states having more individualistic and traditional political cultures—particularly if the moralistic states continue their tendency not to subsidize their university hospitals.

The situation in moralistic states can also be viewed more positively. Their university hospitals may have a competitive advantage by virtue of either their product mix or their differentiation in favor of superspecialty and tertiary-care levels. These hospitals also tend to be more efficient.

The implications of ownership are less clear. All university hospitals will be under increasingly severe financial pressures. First, all of them will be under pressure to fund charity care for the one-third of all persons below the official poverty line who are not covered by Medicaid [18,19]. Private university hospitals will be less able to obtain state subsidies for these costs. Second, there will be intense pressures on accumulating capital funds. Private university hospitals will have the advantage here, because they are freer to form or join hospital corporations that can make stock offerings; public university hospitals will continue to have to borrow under state sponsorship. Private hospitals will be able to obtain more philanthropic gifts, whereas public hospitals will continue to receive state subsidies.

Private hospitals enjoy two more advantages over public hospitals. The first is their more focused, decentralized governance, which can respond quickly to competition because it places power closer to the university hospital and among fewer power holders. In contrast, public university hospitals are usually more centralized and power is shared by many in a multilayered complex decision-making hierarchy. More important perhaps, public university hospitals are tax supported and state owned; they are constrained by state officials from competing fully with the private sector.

The second advantage of private hospitals is their greater superspecialization or product differentiation. Our conclusions here have less support, but we know that private universities and their medical schools depend more on research funds, and this fact implies a greater degree of specialization among their clinical faculty. This specialization is likely to be mirrored partially in the university hospitals' clinical services and patient mix. Although we did not directly measure these two variables, we believe the inference is reasonable.

What is less clear is whether greater specialization is a viable competitive strategy. A university hospital specializing in rare diseases and injuries will have high unit costs but compete with fewer institutions having equally high unit costs. These hospitals will have some monopoly in their regions in such highly specialized areas. Conversely, other hospitals will skim the market by stressing more routine care. They will have high volume and low unit costs, but compete with a much larger number of peer institutions. Thus far there seems to be no clear financial advantage to either of these product strategies. However, if a university hospital were to stress routine care, it would cease to provide a comprehensive clinical laboratory to its medical school, and thus be less useful as a university hospital. The only way this strategy could be pursued is for the medical school to affiliate with nonuniversity hospitals. In this case, the private university hospital would have the advantage in its greater ability to form or join hospital chains like the one formed by Rush-Presbyterian St. Luke's Hospital in Chicago. In that system, outstate hospitals in Illinois provide less specialized care and refer their rarer cases to the base university hospital at Rush. Thus, by virtue of their private ownership per se and their tendency toward specialization, the private university hospitals seem to have some advantage over the public university hospitals. They may be able to adapt better to the environment they are likely to face in the near future.

REFERENCES

1. Pierce, B., and E. Hekman. *Health care cost containment legislation: 1983 legislative update fifty states, Paper #1*. Denver, Colo.: National Conference of State Legislatures, 1984.

2. Allison, R.F., and J. Dalston. Goverance of university-owned teaching hospitals. *Inquiry* 19(1982):3–17.
3. The third study of general manufacturing business climates of the forty-eight contiguous states of America, 1981. Chicago: Alexander Grant & Co. in cooperation with the Conference of State Manufacturers' Associations (COSMA), 1981.
4. Elazar, D.J. *American federalism: A view from the states.* New York: Thomas Y. Crowell Co., 1966, pp. 84–126.
5. Churchman, C.W. *The systems approach.* New York: Dell Publishing Co., 1968, p. 50.
6. Astley, W.G., and A.H. Van de Ven. Central perspectives and debates in organization theory. *Administrative Science Quarterly* 28(1983):245–73.
7. Elazar, *American federalism.*
8. Almond, G.A., and S. Verba. *The civic culture: Political attitudes and democracy in five nations.* Princeton, N.J.: Princeton University Press, 1963.
9. Almond, G.A., and S. Verba. *The civic culture revisited.* Boston: Little, Brown & Co., 1980.
10. Elazar, *American federalism.*
11. Sharkansky, I. The utility of Elazar's political culture. *Policy* 2(1969): 66–83.
12. Johnson, C.A. Political culture in American states: Elazar's formulation examined. *American Journal of Political Science* 20(1976):491–509.
13. Millard, R.M. Power of state coordinating agencies. In *Improving academic management* edited by P. Jedamus and M.W. Peterson. San Francisco: Jossey-Bass Publishers, 1980, pp. 65–95.
14. National Center for Education Statistics. *Digest of education statistics 1980.* Washington, D.C.: U.S. Government Printing Office, 1980, pp. 142, 159.
15. Pierce and Hekman, Legislative update.
16. Mindlin, S.E., and H. Aldrich. Interorganizational dependence: A review of the concept and a reexamination of the findings of the Aston group. *Administrative Science Quarterly* 20(1975):382–92.
17. Zald, M.N. The power and functions of boards of directors: A theoretical synthesis. *American Journal of Sociology* 75(1969):97–111.
18. Rogers, D.E., R.J. Blendon, and T.W. Moloney. Who needs Medicaid? *New England Journal of Medicine* 307(1982):13–18.
19. Iglehart, J.K. Federal policies and the poor. *New England Journal of Medicine* 307(1982):836–40.

SIX

Testing the Limits of the State Environment

This chapter consolidates and expands upon the topics discussed in chapters 3, 4, and 5 so we may carry out a logical next step: that of empirically testing the extent of their effects. If the state environment can be clearly defined and operationalized as being a combination of the competitive (chapter 3) and political environments (chapter 5), hospital performance (chapter 4) and other hospital-related issues can be predicted in part by the nature of that state environment. As should be evident by this statement, we are here testing the joint effects of previously discussed variables in an attempt to assess how a "state environment" affects the hospital and hospital-related matters.

BACKGROUND

Earlier research into the viability of teaching hospitals examined the role of the state and the financial health of the city [1,2]. In general, however, the intricate political and financial environment of hospitals has not received proper analytic attention. As discussed in chapter 5,

---

This chapter contains some material from Choi, T. Systematic impact of the state on CEO tenure. *Health Care Management Review* 9(Summer 1984):81–84. Reprinted with permission of Aspen Systems Corp., copyright 1984.

we underscored and extended the above-mentioned research by identifying the comprehensive state "political environment" that influences the viability of state-owned university hospitals. And in chapter 3 we described the market index, which is a way of measuring the state's "competitive environment."

The combination of the political and competitive environment creates a context that has consequences for hospital performance. That is, the amount of external support the university hospital receives, the extent of regulations the university hospital faces, and the number of competing facilities all pressure the university hospital to behave or perform in certain ways. Hospitals that count on state support are particularly, though not exclusively, susceptible to state influences. Therefore state-owned university hospitals with similar state environments should face similar issues that will result in relatively similar performance levels. As mentioned in the first paragraph of this chapter, if the state environment can be clearly defined and operationalized, *hospital performance can in part be predicted by the nature of the state environment.* That is, hospitals with similar environmental contexts will probably have similar levels of performance. Therefore, the ability to classify hospitals according to their environments is an important step toward predicting hospital viability.

In this chapter we consider the joint influence of the political environment and the competitive environment. For simplicity, we call the political and competitive environment the state environment. But because state competitiveness does not necessarily apply at the local level, we have augmented this measure of state environment with a third variable called "local competition." We hypothesized that the state environment has an impact upon a number of areas critical to the university hospital, namely (1) hospital viability, (2) comprehensiveness of state-subsidized indigent care, and (3) length of CEO tenure.

OPERATIONALIZATION OF VARIABLES

Most of the variables used in this chapter as shown in table 6.1 have been defined and operationalized in earlier chapters. The competitive environment, measured by the market index, is described in chapter 3. The political environment is described in chapter 5. Hospital performance is represented by the variable "hospital viability," which is defined in two ways (with and without appropriations) in chapter 4.

Three variables remain to be defined here: (1) local competition, (2) comprehensiveness of state-subsidized indigent care, and (3) length of CEO tenure.

Table 6.1 State Environment and Hospital Viability

Scores of State Proactivism and Competition	Viability without Appropriations	Viability with Appropriations
High ($\bar{X}$ is based on 6 UHs in these states)	$\bar{X} = -0.12$	$\bar{X} = 0.03$
Medium ($\bar{X}$ is based on 6 UHs in these states)	$\bar{X} = -0.18$	$\bar{X} = -0.01$
Low ($\bar{X}$ is based on 7 UHs in these states)	$\bar{X} = -0.25$	$\bar{X} = -0.07$

The first variable, local competition, is composed of the number of health care facilities in the university hospital's primary service area. These facilities include other teaching hospitals, tertiary care medical centers, county hospitals, multihospital systems, major private-practice medical groups, large HMO practices, and large IPAs (independent practice associations). The correlation between the number of health care facilities and the number of competing hospitals in the same geographical area is 0.53, $p = .001$. We know from this correlation that the number of local health care facilities is directly associated with competition.

The second variable, comprehensiveness of state-subsidized indigent care, is defined by the number of optional Medicaid services above and beyond the required minimum the state provides to those on Medicaid. Recipients include both the categorically needy (people receiving federally supported financial assistance) and the medically needy (people who are eligible for medical but not financial assistance).

The third variable, length of CEO tenure, is measured by the number of years served by a CEO in that capacity at the university hospital. The CEO position is typically held by someone trained as an administrator. In rare occasions the hospital CEO is also a physician from the medical school faculty, or a health science school official, for example the associate vice-president for health affairs.

METHODOLOGY

Classifying University Hospitals by State Environment

In order to test the impact of the state environment, we stratified the states in which university hospitals are located in terms of high, medium, and low scores, in (1) state proactivism (the political environment variable used in chapter 5), (2) state competitiveness (the market index used in chapter 3), and (3) local competition.

University hospitals may score differently—high, medium, or low—in each of the three variables. We discarded from further analyses those hospitals scoring high on one variable but low or medium on others, and retained those hospitals scoring consistently on all three variables—all high scores, or all medium, or all low. For example, a hospital retained for analysis scored "high" on state proactivism (i.e., highly regulated state), state competitiveness (highly competitive state), and local competition. Such consistency provides the most straightforward test of the relationship between type of environment and hospital performance, because the environment type is unquestioned. While states with hybrid scores (e.g., extensive regulation but minimal competition) could have been used as part of this test, their inclusion would have complicated the scoring and unnecessarily obscured the central thesis: that state environment, once it is clearly identified, may be shown to have systematic impact on hospital viability.

FINDINGS

Effects on Viability

Table 6.1 shows the distribution of viability scores of university hospitals grouped according to state proactivism and competition into three groups. The magnitude of score differences between the three groups is not trivial.

Because the individual score for each hospital changes from year to year, hospital scores are aggregated by group. This averages out the effects of an unusual year (a frequent occurrence in university hospital finances), and prevents the individual measures from severely skewing the results.

The nature of the state environment as shown in table 6.1 is clearly associated with hospital viability. The negative values in the first column indicate that none of the three groups of university hospitals is financially solvent without the aid of state appropriations. (In fact, the raw data on which table 6.1 is based show that none of the individual hospitals under the first column is financially solvent without appropriations.) However, hospitals situated in proactive (and wealthier) states tend to fare better, hovering closer to the financial break-even point (mean = -0.12). If the viability measure of total patient-care revenue includes appropriation dollars (second column), hospitals in proactive states still have a relative advantage over hospitals in other states. However, the score improvement is crucial: the appropriation generally helps hospitals in proactive states move into financial solvency (mean = 0.03), whereas the remaining two groups tend to continue to be financially troubled in degrees consistent with the level of state proactivism.

Figure 6.1 corroborates the information provided thus far: that the environment affects performance if only the environment can be clearly defined. Under figure 6.1, three path models are shown. The first model (I) is based on a sample of all university hospitals—public and private—and assesses the impact of the environment on viability (here used without state appropriations). Because the sample includes both public and private university hospitals, the level of dependency of these hospitals on state proactiveness is very mixed (see chapter 5) and not systematic. The results tend to confirm the impact of this deliberate indiscriminate mixing of different levels of state environments and different ownership of hospitals. This path model (I) explains only 16 percent of the variation in viability. The independent variable, state competitiveness, actually shows a positive impact on viability.

The second path model (II) eliminates the private hospitals from analysis. In so doing, the sample is now more homogenized, made up of hospitals that are uniformly more dependent on state proactivism. As would be expected, the impact of state competitiveness in model II turns negative on viability and the relative effect of state proactivism increases greatly. In short, state proactivism serves to protect and help state-owned university hospital viability. It may be interpreted that private university hospitals, relative to their public counterparts, tend to prevail over health care competition.

Finally, the third model (III) is similar to that used in table 6.1, and includes only those university hospitals whose scores on the three environmental variables were consistent (all high, all medium, or all low). By so doing, when the environment is clear and its facets consistent, not only is the portion of the explained variance increased to 26 percent, but the protection and help given by the state also become much clearer and pronounced (path coefficient = .845). The negative impact of state competitiveness is also more crystallized and prominent (path coefficient = −.370).

The results again confirm the impact of the state on state-owned university hospital viability. It is especially evident that when the environment can be clearly defined, its impact is undeniably more pronounced. From these results we can postulate that public university hospital viability follows the nature and type of environment. The

Figure 6.1 Increasing Clarity of Environmental Impact on Hospital Viability

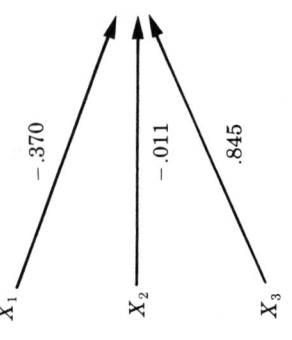

I. Unclear Environment
(State-owned and private UHs, mixed environment score)

$X_1 \xrightarrow{.209} V$
$X_2 \xrightarrow{.062} V$
$X_3 \xrightarrow{.186} V$

$r^2 = .16$

II. Hybrid Environment
(State-owned UHs only, mixed environment score)

$X_1 \xrightarrow{-.037} V$
$X_2 \xrightarrow{.023} V$
$X_3 \xrightarrow{.455} V$

$r^2 = .19$

III. Clear Environment
(State-owned UHs only, consistent environment score)

$X_1 \xrightarrow{-.370} V$
$X_2 \xrightarrow{-.011} V$
$X_3 \xrightarrow{.845} V$

$r^2 = .26$

Note:
X_1 = State competition;
X_2 = Local competition;
X_3 = State proactivism;
V = Viability without appropriation.

results illustrate the dependence of state-owned university hospital on state support and protection.

State Support of Health Care for the Poor

Our second critical issue, the comprehensiveness of indigent care, is explained by table 6.2. This table shows that the comprehensiveness of indigent care varies in direct proportion to state proactivism and competition.

Since university hospitals are often expected to care for the poor, state subsidization of the poor alleviates financial risk for university hospitals. High state proactivism has two clear effects. First, hospitals in highly proactive states can count both on state protection—that is, financial help—and on state coverage of indigent care. Second, highly proactive states are willing to provide broad health care coverage for both the categorically and the medically needy. Because eligibility is less restrictive and coverage more comprehensive, hospitals incur less financial risk when caring for the poor. Less proactive states tend to limit coverage to the categorically needy only; hospitals in those states therefore absorb more costs. A caution should be introduced here, how-

Table 6.2 State Environment and Comprehensiveness of Medicaid Services

	FMAP%*	Additional Services above the Required Minimum Offered by State Medicaid Programs to:		
		CN† Only	CN & MN‡	Total
Highly proactive and competitive states	$\bar{X} = 50.50$	$\bar{X} = 5.50$	$\bar{X} = 18.67$	$\bar{X} = 24.17$
Medium proactive and competitive states	$\bar{X} = 61.17$	$\bar{X} = 6.83$	$\bar{X} = 11.83$	$\bar{X} = 18.67$
Low proactive and competitive states	$\bar{X} = 71.43$	$\bar{X} = 8.14$	$\bar{X} = 8.29$	$\bar{X} = 16.43$
Grand Mean	61.58	6.89	12.68	19.58

Data source: Department of Health and Human Services, Health Care Financing Administration, Office of Intergovernmental Affairs, October 1, 1983.

*Federal Medicaid Percentage (FMAP): Rate of federal financial participation in a state's medical assistance program under Title XIX of the Social Security Act. The lower the percent, the more the state is supplementing.

†Categorically Needy: People receiving federally supported financial assistance.

‡Medically Needy: People who are eligible for medical but not financial assistance.

ever. While proactive states have been willing to underwrite the cost of caring for the indigents at the university hospital, federal efforts in the form of DRGs—standardizing and publicizing reimbursement figures on the basis of typical costs—may make it more difficult for the university hospital to be subsidized at its current levels. That is, while the state is willing to reimburse the university hospital (directly or indirectly) on cost-based service, the federal government is reimbursing on typical case-based service. The dollar disparity between the two, whether due to difference in case-acuity or simply education-induced inefficiencies, would probably raise questions about the cost of care at the university hospital, even if it is situated in a proactive state.

State Environment and CEO Tenure

States that are highly competitive and proactive also have a systematic negative impact on the longevity of CEO tenure at state-owned university hospitals. This impact is not overwhelming, though it is noteworthy. The point here is not to attribute short tenure solely to the nature of the state but to indicate that the state, through other variables (see figure 6.2) contributes to shortening CEO tenure. Our study found that the average CEO tenure in these hospitals is 6.21 years, compared with 9.52 years enjoyed by CEOs in industrial firms [3]. Even more telling is the hospital CEOs' median—vis-à-vis the average—tenure of 5 years. Forty-six percent of state university hospital CEOs served in their present capacity for 4 years or less. This shows that CEOs at university hospitals have shorter tenure, possibly the consequence of the governance and managerial control they lack. This lack of control has been attributed in part to the nature of state ownership [4]. The state's ownership influence contributes to making the job of the university hospital CEO both difficult and unique.

Figure 6.2 shows how a state's competitiveness also simultaneously limits managerial influence. [Managerial influence is measured by the CEO's influence over 6 decisions: (1) reorganizing at the governance level to give substantial autonomy to the university hospital, (2) allocating space within the hospital, (3) establishing personnel policies and procedures, (4) making medical staff appointments, (5) determining staff pay, and (6) determining bed allocations by service. These 6 decisions were identified as a set through factor analysis from among 14 decisions.] Local competition also is shown to reduce managerial influence, which in turn leads to shorter tenure (see figure 6.2). In short, competitiveness at both the state and local level acts to hasten CEO turnover by limiting CEO managerial influence. The direct effect of competition on tenure $(-.029)$ is negligible.

Figure 6.2 Factors Affecting CEO Tenure
(State University Hospitals, $N = 33$)

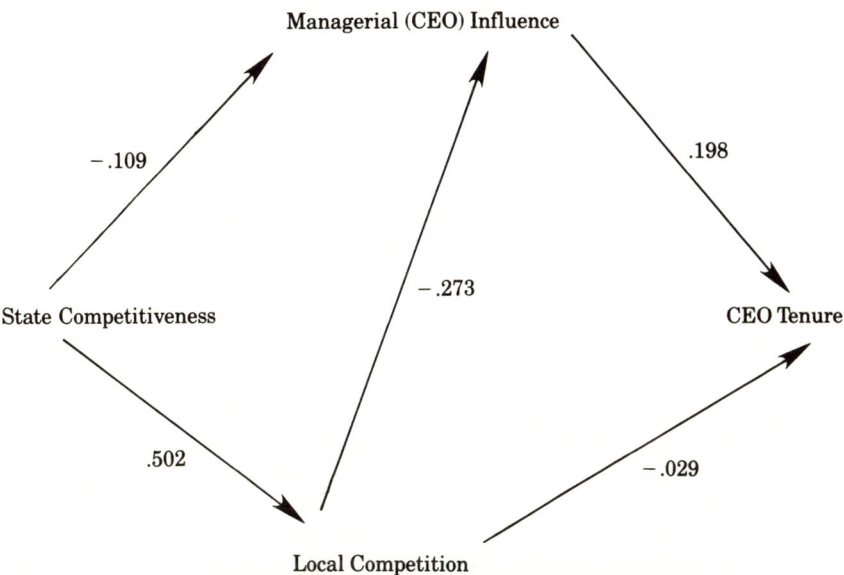

Reprinted, adapted, with permission from *Health Care Management Review* 9(Summer 1984):83.

These results are consistent with current findings that a manager's marginal degree of influence and lack of control over governance and environment play a part in precipitating CEO turnover [3,5]. These reasons for turnover apparently are independent of organizational performance and the hospital's financial viability [3,6].

DISCUSSION

The preceding three sets of results show that when an environment can be clearly identified, hospitals in similar environments tend to have corresponding viability scores. This supports the hypothesis that factors outside the hospital strongly influence viability. These factors are not random; they form a sort of consistent environmental context that has an impact on more than just hospital viability.

However, it is difficult to assess to what extent the state environment directly contributes to hospital viability. It is possible that the state context attracts and promotes a certain type of management and interorganizational relationship, that in turn contributes to hospital viability.

Because of differences in the character of state ownership and state dependency, management effectiveness has to be viewed within the context of the state environment. A manager's success in one university hospital may be the result of a proper mix between the specific skills of that manager and the environmental characteristics of the state. Therefore, to compare managerial effectiveness across disparate state environments would be judging managerial effectiveness on unequal footing. It is unfortunate that it is far easier to blame the hospital CEO than to grapple with state passivity.

What is clear is that the state environment cannot be ignored when assessing hospital viability. It is a step toward realistic hospital governance and management—at least in state-owned university hospitals—to recognize the constraints imposed by the state and to devise appropriate means to deal with these constraints.

IMPLICATIONS FOR MANAGEMENT

What can hospital management do to enhance hospital viability? While there is no panacea, the obvious and, we believe, the correct conclusion is to work as closely as possible with key decision makers in the state. In chapter 2 we referred to university hospitals as protected organizations because the state takes pride in them. To foster and intensify this pride could only help the university hospital and it is incumbent upon the recent generation of hospital administrators and their boards to spearhead this effort. The importance of lobbying state officials applies to both public and private university hospital administrators because some private university hospitals (e.g., in Pennsylvania) are state assisted.

Until recently, history has shown that the health care environment has favored the university hospital. Hospital administrators have been able to make their reputation on internal management. However, the proliferation of competition in advanced tertiary care now renders the university hospital more vulnerable. Competitive pressures have profound effects on university hospital management. A capable manager of internal affairs is no longer sufficient to guarantee hospital stability and viability. Besides, the nature of internal problems to be managed changes as the health care environment changes. Hospital managers are therefore caught in uncertain tides and the traditional routes to managerial success and recognition no longer apply.

Working with key decision makers of the state implies an awareness of what these decision makers require. They need to be able to satisfy their own constituencies. To the extent that the university hospital is able to provide and publicize satisfactory services to such constituencies, it stands a good chance of being continually protected. Because state constituencies are likely to be diverse, the hospital needs to be able to diversify its promotions, products, and services. Such diversity may not always be feasible; in that case the hospital needs to match, to the degree possible, its feasible products with the critical constituencies. While this implies setting priorities for certain departments, products, and services—which can never be done without generating waves of political conflict—it may be a necessary step to improve hospital viability.

Working with external decision makers also implies a governance and management change within the university hospital. The hospital will need a governance group that represents the hospital extensively and intensively. This will usually mean a departure from the traditional methods of governance. The new governance requires a board that is intimately aware of the external and internal pressures faced by the university hospital, and willing to represent the hospital in appealing for support. The allocation of authority to hospital administration or its representatives to speak for the hospital may require reorganization at both the university and hospital levels.

At the university level, the university board of trustees or a subcommittee of the board will either have to take a more active role in the hospital governance or be willing to delegate the governance role to another group. Dilution of trustee authority is not a minor matter, the consideration of which is usually fraught with dissension.

At the hospital level, an administration that must pay increasing attention to the environment and the hospital board will need to delegate many of the internal management duties to other administrators. This transition would require an organizational change (for example, decentralization) which, if attempted, is usually accompanied by at least some prerequisite reorganizational pains.

Lobbying state officials is not easy; it requires that the hospital speak with a relatively unified voice. Unanimity of opinions has not traditionally been endemic to the university. Hospital administrators and their boards will need to galvanize the many parties associated with the hospital and raise their awareness regarding the need to seek state protection and the need for the hospital to be represented with singularity and authority. Hospital administrators may need to take risks when necessary in working with state officials to set forth a probable hospital position when none has been forged.

Competitive pressures may justify more radical organizational changes. In less proactive states where university hospitals are less protected by their owners, more extensive corporate restructuring might be necessary. That is, unless the university or the state takes ownership of the hospital, the hospital might be better able to thrive as a separate corporation, either with a for-profit or nonprofit status. If it is nonprofit, the hospital may appeal to the state or other benefactors directly rather than through the university. If it is for-profit, then market pressures may force some hospitals to trim their teaching and research commitments. At this writing only one university hospital has taken the route of separate incorporation, and subsequent hospital viability was improved.

So far, the strategies described differ for hospitals in proactive and nonproactive states. But a strategy that applies equally to all hospitals is that of forming linkages with other hospitals or health care–related organizations. Establishing relationships with competing organizations has the advantage of potentially stablizing the market. It is feasible that interdepartmental cooperation on some services between hospitals may save costs and improve the teaching and research functions. Although the likelihood of this kind of cooperation is not overwhelming, establishing a means of interhospital communication makes it possible to cooperate if and when cooperation is warranted. It could be attempted first on a small scale, as in joint purchasing of necessary products and services. The discounts available to all hospitals from such ventures make it a no-lose situation. (Some university hospitals may be in a better position to cooperate with other university hospitals across state lines than with hospitals in the immediate region.)

In any event current market pressures demand that the university hospital administration pay more attention to the hospital environment than ever before. Appealing to the state for support, changing the governance structure, delegating internal management to lower level administrators, making the hospital a corporation separate from the university, and forming ties with other health care organizations are all means of dealing with a changing environment. In the next chapter we will further demonstrate the need for hospital administrators to focus their efforts on the environment by showing the impact of environment on hospital performance.

REFERENCES

1. Schramm, C.J. The teaching hospital and the future role of state government. *New England Journal of Medicine* 308(1983):41–45.
2. Hadley, J., R. Mullner, and J. Feder. The financially distressed hospital. *New England Journal of Medicine* 307(1982):1283–87.
3. Allen, M.P., and S.K. Panian. Power, performance, and succession in the large corporation. *Administrative Science Quarterly* 27(1982):538–47.
4. Kinzer, D.M. Turnover of hospital chief executive officers: A hospital association perspective. *Hospital and Health Services Administration* 27(1982): 11–33.
5. Pfeffer, J., and G.R. Salancik. Organizational context and the characteristics and tenure of hospital administrators. *Academy of Management Journal* 20(1977):74–88.
6. See chap. 7.

SEVEN

The Impact of the Environment on University Hospital Performance: An Explanatory Model

In chapters 2 through 6 we defined, correlated, and analyzed a multitude of variables. In this chapter we sequence a number of these variables in a model to examine the systematic relationship between a university hospital and its environment. Our definition of "environment" has been enlarged as we progressed; it has also proven to be increasingly complex.

Is it possible to construct an open-systems model of state-owned university hospitals—one that identifies the sequence of factors contributing to their governance, management, and performance? This is the task we have set for ourselves in this chapter. Because we are entering uncharted territory, the path model described in this chapter should be viewed as exploratory.

The path model began as a basic conceptual model shown in figure 2.1 of chapter 2. We expanded this in figure 2.2 and again now into the path model shown in figure 7.1. Figure 7.1 includes ten environmental and organizational variables, and two types of performance

---

This chapter is an adapted version of "Impact of Environment on State University Hospital Performance," *Medical Care* 23(July 1985):855–71. Reprinted with permission.

Figure 7.1 Hypotheses

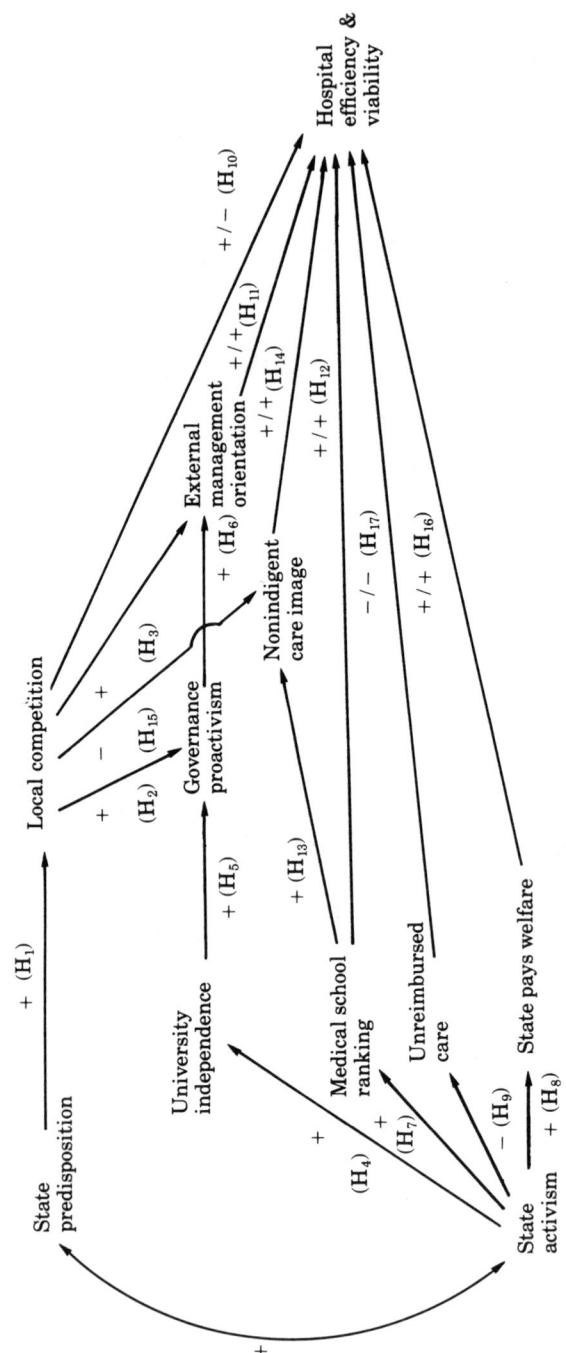

Reprinted with permission from *Medical Care* 23(July 1985):857.

Notes:
+ Denotes a hypothesized positive relationship.
− Denotes a hypothesized negative relationship.
+/− Denotes a hypothesized positive relationship for efficiency but a negative relationship for viability.

outcome: efficiency and viability. The relationships between the above variables constitute 17 hypotheses that would be tested.

The hypotheses in figure 7.1 are designated by abbreviations (H_1, H_2, etc.). The plus and minus signs indicate the hypothesized positive or negative relationship between variables; a double sign ($+/-$, or $+/+$, or $-/-$) occurs next to the hypotheses that lead directly to the outcome or dependent variable "hospital efficiency and viability." These split signs denote one hypothesized effect on efficiency (first sign) and another hypothesized effect on viability (second sign).

We used the path analysis method to test our hypothesis; this method has been explained in chapter 2 and will not be repeated here. Our explanation of the variables used in the path model is found in the next section. The basic statistics for these variables are shown in table 7.1.

Table 7.1 Frequency Distribution of Variables in the Path Model

Variable	N	$\bar{X}$	Standard Deviation	Range
1. State predisposition*	34	4.34	2.04	0.00 to 7.54
2. State activism*	34	−0.09	0.90	−1.34 to 1.24
3. Local competition*	34	0.02	0.85	−1.41 to 2.17
4. University independence*	34	−0.16	0.58	−1.13 to 1.89
5. Medical school ranking	33	55.52	30.47	5.00 to 106.00
6a. Appropriations	34	0.16	0.11	0.00 to 0.44
6b. Unreimbursed care	33	17.73	13.22	3.00 to 45.00
7. State pays welfare	34	135.53	69.82	35.00 to 294.00
8. Nonindigent care image*	34	−0.14	0.78	−1.89 to 1.54
9. Governance proactivism	34	0.94	1.72	0.00 to 9.00
10. External management orientation*	34	−0.14	1.36	−2.30 to 4.66
11. Efficiency*	34	−0.30	0.78	−2.14 to 1.25
12. Viability	32	−0.16	0.12	−0.48 to 0.08

Reprinted with permission from *Medical Care* 23(July 1985):858.
*Signifies Z-standardization of variables in index.

HYPOTHESES AND RATIONALE

The following hypotheses are stated in axiomatic form, consistent with the path model (see figure 7.1). A brief rationale follows and justifies each hypothesis based on literature support, information from field interviews, and logical internal consistency with the rest of the statements in the model.

1. The greater the degree of state competitiveness, the more competing facilities there will be in the local environment.
   Rationale: Logical deduction.
2. The more competing facilities there are in the university hospital's service area, the more proactive the governing board will be.
   Rationale: Organizations subject to external influence select board members who take initiative to help the organization deal with the environment [1,2].
3. The more competing facilities there are, the more externally oriented management will be.
   Rationale: Logical consistency with hypothesis 2. External competition forces management to pay attention to the environment.
4. The more proactive the state, the more independent the university will be.
   Rationale: High state proactivism indicates a state that emphasizes health, education, and welfare. Strong emphasis in education reflects concomitant stress on research, which in turn generates nonstate research funding and helps the university become less state dependent.
5. The more independent the university, the more proactive the governance of the hospital will be.
   Rationale: University independence generates independence for its units. (Governance may be provided by a special board appointed by the regents or by the regents themselves. The point is not who governs, but how proactive governance is. Therefore, our operationalization of this variable centers on proactivity, not on the governing body.)
6. The more proactive the governance, the more externally oriented management will be.
   Rationale: Governance proactivism implies being proactive with the hospital environment. It is logical to hypothesize

that a governing board with a proactive bent is likely to have a hospital management with the same orientation. External orientation is a response to environmental uncertainties, as evidenced by university hospitals establishing hospital-specific governing boards to help management better deal with the competitive environment.

7. The more proactive the state, the higher the ranking of the medical school will be.
Rationale: State proactivism is expected to emphasize education [3].

8. The more proactive the state, the more welfare it pays (removing the burden of unreimbursed care from the university hospital).
Rationale: Proactive states characteristically place heavy emphasis on assuming welfare responsibilities [4].

9. The more proactive the state, the less it will make direct appropriations or give unreimbursed care dollars to the hospital.
Rationale: This is consistent with hypothesis 8 and its rationale. A proactive state is less likely to make appropriations directly to a hospital when such appropriations in the form of welfare or health care reimbursement have been made to the patient.

10a. The more competing facilities there are, the better the hospital efficiency will be.
Rationale: Competition encourages efficiency.

10b. The more competing facilities there are, the more precarious the hospital's viability will be.
Rationale: Extreme competition tends to deplete health care dollars. University hospitals, by virtue of their multiple missions and costly tertiary care, are likely to become less viable in highly competitive settings where profits depend on highly streamlined services unencumbered by teaching and research costs.

11. The more externally oriented the management, the better the hospital will perform.
Rationale: This is consistent with current organizational theory, and assumes that modern complex organizations are very vulnerable to external influences. Management that looks externally will be in a better position to respond internally and to survive [5].

12. The higher the medical school ranking, the better the university hospital performance will be.
    Rationale: Logical deduction. University hospitals are staffed by medical school faculty and residents; the quality and reputation of the medical school are expected to help hospital performance.
13. The higher the medical school ranking, the less the university hospital will be seen as a place for indigent or charity care.
    Rationale: Some university hospitals accept a disproportionate amount of indigent or charity care patients [6]. This perceived negative image drives away some patients who are more able to pay. The image, whether justified or not, may be offset by a medical school with a sterling reputation; the hospital may then be seen as a place for quality care, regardless of the social and economic characteristics of some of its patients.
14. The less the hospital is seen as an indigent care center, the more efficient and viable the hospital.
    Rationale: Low visibility as indigent care center will enable attraction of paying patients. This should help the hospital to be more competitive.
15. The more competing facilities there are, the more likely the university hospital will have an indigent care image.
    Rationale: Since a state university hospital is directly or indirectly supported by the state, it seems a logical place for indigents to go, often with encouragement from competing hospitals. Moreover the university hospital's location, often in or close to the inner city, encourages the patronage of the many indigents likely to reside there.
16. The more the state pays in welfare, the greater the viability and the lower the efficiency of the university hospital will be.
    Rationale: Logical reasoning: if the state does not pay for indigent care in all hospitals, this financial burden will be assumed disproportionately by university hospitals. Therefore, a state that pays welfare helps university hospital viability but reduces the incentive for efficiency [6].
17. The more the state appropriates funds or reimburses the hospital for indigent care, the worse the performance of university hospitals will be.
    Rationale: Particularly in hospitals that receive state appro-

priation based on need, the incentive for efficiency is reduced (same rationale for hypothesis 16).

VARIABLES, SCALES, AND SCALE ITEMS USED IN THE PATH MODEL

1. State competitiveness (scale reliability, using Cronbach's alpha = 0.91), composed of three indexes already explained in chapter 3:
   A. Per capita income within state
   B. Percent of urbanization within state
   C. Ratio of medical specialists to population
2. State proactivism (scale reliability, using Cronbach's alpha = 0.91), composed of four existing scales; is expanded here from chapters 3 and 5:
   A. Political culture scale [7]
   B. Legislative innovativeness scale [8]
   C. Legislative organizational effectiveness ranking [4]
   D. Redistribution of income to the poor [9]
   Note: a socially and legislatively active state is expected to emphasize and support health, education and welfare.
3. Number of competing facilities in the university hospital's self-defined service area (abbreviated as local competition), composed of:
   A. Number and variety of major competing facilities. Data were obtained through the following means: each CEO of each university hospital was asked the following questions [10]:
      1. How many hospitals are there in your primary service area?
      2. How many hospitals in your primary service area would you consider to be competitive?
      3. How many of the following facilities are available in your primary service area?
         a. Teaching hospitals
         b. Tertiary care medical centers
         c. County hospitals
         d. Multihospital systems
         e. Major private practice medical groups (who depend on referrals)
         f. Large HMO practice
         g. Large IPAs
   Each "yes" answer for 3a through 3g was given 1 point. Total points were summed across the seven items. The index, com-

106 / *Governing University Hospitals*

posed of items 1, 2, and 3, yielded a Cronbach's alpha of 0.72. A scale score is computed for each hospital.

4. University financial independence (abbreviated as university independence [scale reliability, using Cronbach's alpha = 0.75]), composed of:
   A. Research expense per FTE at the university in 1981
   B. Total educational and general expenditure per FTE in 1981
   C. State/local appropriation as percent of total university revenue in 1981 (reversed for scaling)
   D. Revenue from government grants and contracts as percent of total revenue in 1981
   E. Research expense as percent of total expenditure in 1981
5. Medical school ranking, composed of the following existent data:
   A. Medical school ranking [11]
6a. Appropriations to hospital, 1981–82, expressed as a proportion of total operating revenue [10] (used only in figure 7.2)
6b. Unreimbursed care, expressed as a proportion of total care delivered (used only in figure 7.3)
7. State/local public welfare burden index (abbreviated as "state pays welfare") state census data, 1977
8. Nonindigent image in community and confidence in attracting nonindigent patients (abbreviated as "nonindigent care image"). Each CEO of each university hospital was asked if the hospital (a) is seen as a place for indigent care, and conversely, (b) will attract all the ambulatory patients it wants, (c) will attract all the normal care inpatients it wants, and (d) will attract all the tertiary care patients it wants.
9. Governance proactivism, explained in table 3.9. The extent to which the governing body initiates governance action (versus merely endorsing proposals).
10. External management orientation: the amount of high level administrative attention paid to:
    A. Third party reimbursement
    B. Regulations
    C. Better health care organizations
    Each CEO of each university hospital was asked the amount of attention paid to specific examples of the above items. Responses were factor analyzed and like items were selected to form this index. An index score was calculated for each hospital.
11. Efficiency, an index explained in chapter 2, Methodology, and composed of:
    A. Inventory value per average daily census, 1981

B. Average days' revenues in receivables, 1981
C. Growth adjusted occupancy, 1979–81 [10] (see chapter 2)
12. Viability, composed of 1980–81 net revenues less state appropriations, expressed as a proportion of 1980–81 total operating expenses [10] (see chapter 2).

RESULTS

As figures 7.2 (efficiency) and 7.3 (viability) show, most hypotheses are supported. The hypotheses not substantiated are: 2, 5, 12, and 15. Essentially, the substance of the two figures shows that political and economic conditions of the state have systematic effects on the independence, governance, and management of the university hospital and on the quality of its performance. A proactive state helps the efficiency and the viability of the university hospital by assuming the health care costs for indigents. Conversely, as expected, such a state also withholds direct appropriations from the university hospital, because these appropriations are likely to be made indirectly through welfare recipients.

Strong state competitiveness also brings intense local competition, which in turn forces university hospitals to be efficient (.293), but the same competition hurts their viability (−.060) though at a statistically insignificant level. Similarly, intense local competition also has an effect, minor though it appears to be (.067), of turning the attention of management outward. An externally oriented management is shown to have a positive impact on hospital efficiency (.305). Intense local competition has two unexpected effects worth noting. It places limits on governing board proactivism, and it does not seem to create an indigent care image for the university hospital (hypotheses 2 and 15).

The second unexpected result concerns the impact of medical school prestige. Although medical school prestige does improve hospital viability, it also reduces efficiency, though almost at a negligible level (−.085). Its influence on hospital indigent care image is minimal (hypothesis 13).

DISCUSSION

In our interviews, some university hospital administrators conveyed the fear that as the health care environment becomes more competitive, university hospitals may increasingly become receptacles for

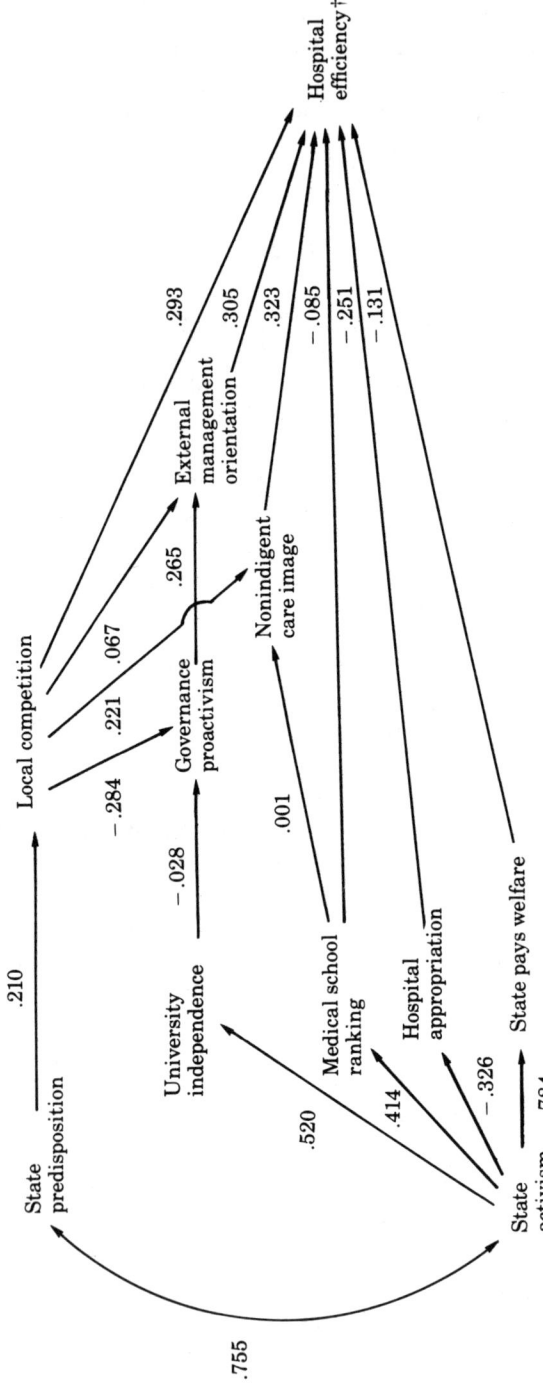

Figure 7.2 Impact of Environment, Governance, and Management on Efficiency (*N* = 34*)

Reprinted with permission from *Medical Care* 23(July 1985):859.
*All coefficients are expected to be generalizable to the population of state university hospitals because sample *N* approximates population.
†Variance explained = 37 percent.

Figure 7.3 Impact of Environment, Governance, and Management on Viability ($N = 34$*)

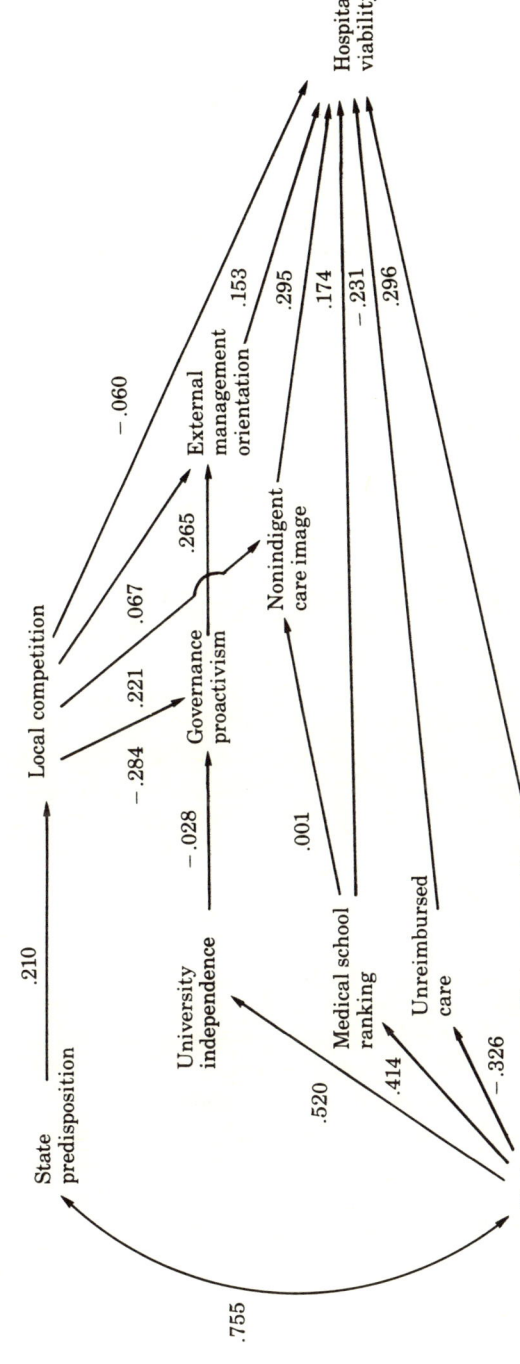

Reprinted with permission from *Medical Care* 23(July 1985):860.

*All coefficients are expected to be generalizable to the population of state university hospitals because sample N approximates population.

†Variance explained = 46 percent.

indigents. This fear was raised by their observations of the current federal administration's fiscal policies, particularly the reduction of welfare support for the poor, resulting in a probable under-reimbursement for health care. Because most university hospitals are state owned, their options regarding indigent care are relatively limited. A hospital with an indigent care image may drive away those image-conscious patients who are able to pay, sending them to competitors.

Results shown in figures 7.2 and 7.3 do not support this fear of "indigent dumping." This is not to say that indigent transfer has not taken place in some settings, and the data do support the proposition that a nonindigent image helps performance. Nevertheless the data indicate that on the whole, intense local competition has not resulted in the university hospital receiving an indigent care image. The indigent transfers that have occurred have not altered the image of the university hospital. We can suggest several explanations for this unexpected finding. First of all, some university hospitals are not situated in indigent population centers, so responses from these hospitals would moderate the impact of indigent transfer. Secondly, it is likely that in addition to the university hospital, nonuniversity teaching and county hospitals also receive indigent transfers. Thus, indigent transfer is somewhat diffused. Thirdly, university hospitals may also be perceived as tertiary care centers. Therefore, even with a heavy indigent care load, their image is not exclusively that of indigent care. None of these probable explanations would adequately reflect the facts of individual settings. As mentioned, however, intensifying competition on the national scale has not made university hospitals indigent care centers.

Local competition appears to be spurring university hospitals into greater efficiency (.293, figure 7.2). Similarly, externally oriented managements seem to have found a better way to respond to the environment by delegating to subordinates the responsibility for internal hospital affairs. This may account for the positive relationship between external orientation and internal efficiency (.305). Both a nonindigent care image and a state that pays welfare are shown to help the university hospital (.295 and .296). The reason appears straightforward. The hospitals are properly reimbursed for care rendered.

It should be noted, however, that efficiency is multifaceted. As used above, efficiency only covers hardware and material, not personnel. We would not expect that efficiency in the nonpersonnel area necessarily generalizes to the personnel domain, because the efficiency in personnel per bed, for example, is complicated by factors such as patient case mix and acuity.

Intense local competition has a negative effect on how proactive the governing board can be ($-.284$). This coefficient indicates that a competitive environment actually usurps governance proactivism. The finding may be explained by the politics of the university and state. As local competition increases, taxpaying competitors make it difficult—by legislative and other restraining processes—for tax-subsidized university hospitals to compete. Restrictions in funding, bed expansion, and capital acquisitions are examples. The agendas of governance are therefore affected by external factors. When external constraints are imposed, hospital governance is forced to be reactive, "putting out fires" rather than generating proactive organizational strategies.

It should be noted that a highly competitive environment also has a very slight negative impact on university hospital viability ($-.060$, figure 7.3). This does not mean that the university hospital cannot compete or is destined to fail. It may be argued that the multiple missions of the university hospital subsidized by patient dollars render the hospital less able to be cost competitive. The options then are to emphasize patient care at the expense of other missions or to find additional appropriations. The first option is less desirable than the second, and in fact the second option is more often sought.

If competition does not help viability, other factors do. As figure 7.3 shows, an externally oriented management helps viability (.153), as does a nonindigent care image (.295) and a highly ranked medical school (.174).

It is reasonable to believe that there are complex relations between environmental competition and hospital viability not fully captured by our analysis. A clear possibility exists that the purpose of competition between health care organizations is not to eliminate the university hospital but to maintain turf. University hospitals may actually serve their competitors by providing appropriation-subsidized care for the underinsured, taking the acute and expensive cases, and introducing new technology to the health care community. If so, to weaken university hospitals would hurt other health care facilities: there is interdependence as well as competition among the service area providers. The competition does not Balkanize the market but stabilizes it.

It may also be postulated that the higher the number of competing facilities, the more resources the service area is likely to have; this abundance should help the viability of all health care facilities including the university hospital. Finally the high number of competing facilities in a service area (as it was defined by the university hospital's administrator) may simply reflect a large service area; this large domain should help viability.

Hospital viability is enhanced (.174, figure 7.3) and efficiency is very slightly compromised ($-.085$, figure 7.2) by the university hospital's teaching mission. These results indicate the overall benefit of a ranking medical school to the university hospital: it helps hospital viability and induces minimal (statistically insignificant) hospital inefficiency. Education and research costs of a high ranking medical school do not appear to hurt university hospital performance.

Some state rules and practices actually discourage state university hospitals from being cost efficient. Several, for example, are forbidden to have a year-end surplus, which creates a disincentive for efficiency. Others, when there is year-end deficit, are reimbursed by the state or through the university. Again, the incentive and mechanism for efficiency are compromised.

The negative relationship between hospital appropriations and both efficiency and viability shows that the corporate form and the ownership of the state university hospital limit the hospital's ability to compete. Reliance on state appropriations in essence makes the state the quasi stockholder of the university and the university hospital. Because of this, university hospitals do not have free license to wage full-fledged competition.

The governance structure of the university hospital has not helped the hospital to compete effectively. Traditionally the governance function has been assumed by the university board of regents, which oversees both academic units and the university hospital. The difference in these two types of units highlights the demand for very different approaches in the philosophy and operations of governance. Fragmentation of attention and remote governance preclude the likelihood of proactive governance and timely response to competition. A change in structure is never without a substantial power struggle and the final compromise never seems fully satisfying to any or all of the parties nor anticipated by them.

As competitive health care facilities proliferate, the traditional monopolistic dominance of university hospitals has often boomeranged into less subtle town and gown conflicts. The lag in adjustment by university hospital personnel to current competitive realities creates a dinosaur effect on the once all-powerful university hospital.

These are some of the factors that reduce the ability of the university hospitals to compete. But some of them can be changed, as indicated by the relatively low value of many of the path coefficients in figures 7.2 and 7.3. One should not assume that a competitive environment is either deterministic or ominously threatening. University hospitals could cultivate sponsorship from the state and appeal to it for help.

Contrary to some management perspectives, competition is not necessarily a debilitating force. The data would support the notion that a setting characterized by high competition has relatively abundant resources. University hospitals in such a setting, therefore, may actually have a built-in financial advantage. The presence of competition may also denote an area that is culturally, financially, and personally appealing. Noncompetitive states may actually be relatively barren of resources. Therefore, the absence of competition may not be construed as a sign of comfort and vitality.

CONCLUSIONS

Currently, the "diagnosis related group" (DRG) prospective-payment system for Medicare patients is being implemented throughout the country. The effect of this system on university hospitals is unknown, but the concept and current implementation have not, by any means, been enthusiastically embraced by university hospitals. Since the current prospective-payment system reimburses hospitals on the basis of type of illness, university hospitals stand to be under-reimbursed for treating patients with high illness severity within a specific diagnostic group. Similarly, since the university hospitals provide tertiary care, some of these illnesses defy single classification or any classification. The adequacy of payment for these illnesses remains to be seen.

It is possible that those patient cases that consume more hospital resources than the payment allows will be referred to other facilities. Since these patients are probably acutely ill with multiple problems, the university hospital is a likely candidate to serve them. It is also possible, under this new payment mechanism, that referrals between formerly competing facilities will become more cooperative. Hospitals will refer to the university hospital patients they are not efficiently equipped to handle.

What the era of prospective payment brings to the viability of the university hospitals remains to be seen. It is clear, however, that with or without prospective payment, cost competition without additional subsidy will put a number of university hospitals—because of their unique mission—at a disadvantage. If not ameliorated, this disadvantage will have consequences on society as well.

From a theoretical perspective, if university hospitals are treated as commercial for-profit organizations, then their destinies are extremely circumscribed in an era of resource competition. However, if university hospitals are treated as not-for-profit organizations protected by their states, then many of them will probably be insulated from financial failure. Again, the amount of insulation for a university hospital differs from state to state. Those states rated high on activism will probably provide greater insulation against financial loss because of the states' tradition and wealth. Hospitals in less active states are less protected.

All three of the theoretical vantage points—resource dependence, population ecology, and protected institutions—are relevant to understanding state-owned university hospitals. The pressures for acquiring needed organizational resources and the genuine fear on the part of hospital administrators of organizational demise in an increasingly competitive health care market instigate a strong movement to change the governance and management structure of public university hospitals. Consequently, a number of such hospitals have boards of trustees appointed solely to govern the university hospitals—a very different arrangement from the traditional regental governance. To the extent that the university hospital is seen as a source of symbolic pride by its owners (i.e., the state, the university, the citizenry), its demise is greatly exaggerated. Thus, the pressures of resource acquisition and competition are real for public university hospitals, as they are for for-profit organizations; but unlike commercial organizations, public university hospitals stand a decidedly better chance of being protected as public institutions.

Implications

Some of the results deserve particular emphasis. How a medical school is ranked appears to have very little impact on hospital efficiency. This may be taken to mean that the medical faculty's research and teaching—which provided the bases for medical school ranking—decreased hospital efficiency only slightly. On the other hand, a high-ranking medical school helps the financial viability of the hospital substantially. This also means that a low-ranking medical school hurts the financial viability of the hospital. One implication is that the missions of research and teaching are not automatically deleterious to university hospital performance.

Secondly, the nature of the state environment is very important to university hospital performance. Decisions made at the state level have clear and documentable impact on hospital performance. It is a point that may prove useful for state officials to know, as they are in positions that could maximize the state's assistance to the university hospital.

In states where emphasis is placed on competition without subsidization, some university hospitals may be justified in considering separate incorporation. The rationale for this is that if a public hospital has to act like a commercial hospital in order to survive, it may need to be structured, governed, and managed like a commercial enterprise.

These are, of course, weighty and complex decisions. Nevertheless, the findings presented in this chapter demand an awareness of such a possibility.

REFERENCES

1. Pfeffer, J. Size, composition, and function of hospital boards of directors: A study of organization-environment linkage. *Administrative Science Quarterly* 18(1973):349–64.
2. Price, J.L. The impact of governing boards on organizational effectiveness and morale. *Administrative Science Quarterly* 8(1963):361–78.
3. Millard, R.M. Power of state coordinating agencies. In *Improving Academic Management* edited by P. Jedamus and M.W. Peterson. San Francisco: Jossey-Bass, Inc., Publishers, 1980, pp. 65–95.
4. Jacob, H., and K.N. Vines, eds. *Politics in the American states*. Boston: Little, Brown & Co., 1969, p. 193.
5. Pfeffer J., and G.R. Salancik. *The external control of organizations*. New York: Harper and Row, 1978.
6. Schramm, C.J. The teaching hospital and the future role of state government. *New England Journal of Medicine* 308(1983):41–45.
7. Sharkansky, I. The utility of Elazar's political culture. *Policy* 2(1969):66–83.
8. Gray, V. Innovation in the states: A diffusion study. *American Political Science Review* 67(1973):1174–85.
9. Booms, B.H., and J.R. Halldorson. The politics of redistribution: A reformulation. *American Political Science Review* 3(1973):924–33.
10. Isaacs, J. *COTH survey of university-owned teaching hospitals' financial and general operating data. 1979, 1980, 1981*. Washington, D.C.: Department of Teaching Hospitals, Association of American Medical Colleges, 1981, 1982, 1983.
11. Gourman, J. *A rating of graduate and professional programs in American and international universities*. Los Angeles: National Education Standards, 1980.

EIGHT

The Financial Viability of University-Owned Hospitals

Our explanatory model in chapter 7 focused on the sequence of factors that may influence or determine a university hospital's efficiency and viability. The measures of viability we used there were relatively simple. In this chapter we use another path model to focus on three specific dimensions of financial viability (not to be confused with the general viability measure we used in the path model in chapter 7). That is, we examine both the hospitals' current financial position and their current performance, which together will determine their future position.

By identifying the characteristics associated with financial viability and by examining the relationships between them, we hope to provide at least some preliminary answers to these questions: Should university hospitals strive to be more competitive? Should university hospitals seek more financial support from the state, and give up some autonomy? Would reduced or increased size increase viability? Are there problems in the area of pricing that affect viability? Should university hospitals change some fundamental elements of their nature, for example, reduce the level of indigent care or decrease the amount of teaching activity? If the governing bodies granted management more influence and autonomy, would viability improve?

BACKGROUND

The finance-related literature on university hospitals has focused on two issues. First, the nature and extent of the effects of teaching and case mix on utilization and costs; second, more recently, the future of university-owned hospitals. Studies have shown that teaching status of hospitals is related to increased costs and utilization, particularly in ancillary areas [1,2,3], but that when case mix or severity of illness is held constant, the cost difference attributable to teaching has been greatly reduced [4]. The differences in case mix between teaching and nonteaching hospitals have been found to be sufficient to generate higher costs per patient in teaching hospitals even if case mix were the only factor [5]. Thus, our evolving picture of teaching hospitals is characterized by higher costs and higher utilization of ancillary services, such as longer length of stay due to the effects of teaching, and a more severe case mix.

There are further characteristics applicable to university hospitals in particular. One midwestern university hospital was found to have a higher medically indigent patient load, larger and more diverse outpatient clinics, lower occupancy, more diagnostic testing, and higher nursing staffing expense (more nurses per bed and more nurses in administrative areas) than comparable nonteaching hospitals [6].

For the past decade the Council of Teaching Hospitals of the Association of American Medical Colleges has been collecting financial and general operating data from university-owned hospitals on an annual basis. Approximately 70 percent of the hospitals reported receiving some state appropriations in fiscal 1979 and 1980. These appropriations represented close to 18 percent of patient revenue, and were the second leading source of revenue behind Medicare (23.5 percent) for those hospitals that received appropriations in 1980. Medicaid provided about 13 percent of net patient revenue, with Blue Cross and commercial insurers representing equal amounts [7]. However, state governmental support of construction has declined over the past decade as well as philanthropic support, with hospitals showing a dramatic shift to debt financing for construction projects [8]. The nature and extent of state government financial involvement in university hospitals is changing.

University hospitals operate in the same arena of health care delivery as other types of specialty referral centers (SRCs): major multispecialty group practices and medical school affiliated hospitals. These SRCs face the same problems but also represent problems for each other in the form of competition. According to Penchansky and Steinhauer, their responses have included specialization within specialization, increased involvement in primary care, development of institutional alliances, traplining and involvement in patient transport [9].

In his article, "A Requiem for the University Hospital," Westerman describes the evolution of university-owned hospitals and suggests that although their problems recently appeared manageable, time may be running out for these "complex, frustrating organizations." He proposes that universities—40-hour, 5-days-per-week educational organizations—might best stay in the hospital business by getting out of the operation and management of 24-hour, 7-days-per-week patient care systems by allowing the hospital far greater autonomy or allowing some other entity to manage it [10].

On the other hand, Schramm has suggested that teaching hospitals will never be in a position to develop a competitive strategy due to their disproportionate burden of indigent care and the effects of teaching upon their prices. Thus, he believes that since state-level governmental interest in hospitals will increase, teaching hospitals should view these developments in a positive light as an opportunity to seek experimental, creative financing mechanisms to ease their fiscal crisis [11].

Although research in university hospitals has not been specifically mentioned in this review of the literature, evidence of involvement in this area can be seen in the annual report of any university hospital, where the latest technological achievements are proudly described. Thus, university hospitals can be characterized by their activities in research, education, indigent care, unique governance and ownership status. In addition, their medical staff structure is unlike that of community hospitals, often being the clinical faculty of the medical school.

These university hospitals are now faced with a less plentiful environment than that to which they have been accustomed. This environment consists of continuing technological advances and their related costs on the production side, and increased scarcity on the revenue side. The hospitals face increased constraints in reimbursement policies, reduced support for teaching, research, and indigent care and increased competition for "desirable" patients. Inherent in these problems is a need for subsidization of certain activities while at the same time there are increased constraints on the ability to cross subsidize.

DETERMINANTS OF UNIVERSITY HOSPITAL FINANCIAL VIABILITY: A MODEL

Figure 8.1 depicts a model of the characteristics hypothesized to affect a university hospital's financial viability, and the hypothesized relationships between them. They include environmental characterictics (the "demand" box in the upper left) and hospital characteristics (the variables ranging along the bottom and middle), as well as utilization characteristics (upper left-center). The relationships between them affect three measures of financial viability (right side): occupancy (use of capacity), profitability (operating margin), and capital structure (ratio of long-term debt to fixed assets). In this section we will discuss each of these characteristics in more detail.

University hospital patients can be classified in different ways, as shown in the utilization box in figure 8.1. These types can be differentiated simply by their case mix or severity of illness, the number of indigent patients, and the pay source of those who can pay for their care. For a hospital of given capacity and price structure, utilization will be determined by the market demand for the hospital's services. We hypothesized that a number of factors determine the shape of this demand. As figure 8.1 shows, these factors include the size of the population, its level of income, its health status, and the type and level of insurance coverage in the population. Furthermore, the number of other facilities in the area providing similar services determines the level of competition for those patients and thus the number who receive care at the university hospital.

Where a patient is hospitalized is usually the physician's decision. Thus physician referral patterns and admitting privileges play a major role in the number and type of patients admitted to a university hospital.

What directly affects the hospital's costs? The first hypothesis is utilization, due both to the number of patients and the type of care they require. Second is the level of education in the institution, which will contribute directly to costs through increases in salaries and other costs of education, and indirectly through the increased use of certain hospital services by interns and residents as part of their learning experience. Third is the level of research carried out in the hospital, which will probably affect costs in a manner similar to education. Fourth is the prices a hospital must pay for wages. That is, costs will be greater in a high-wage-level area than in an area with lower wage levels.

A fifth hypothesized factor is the size of the hospital. Obviously,

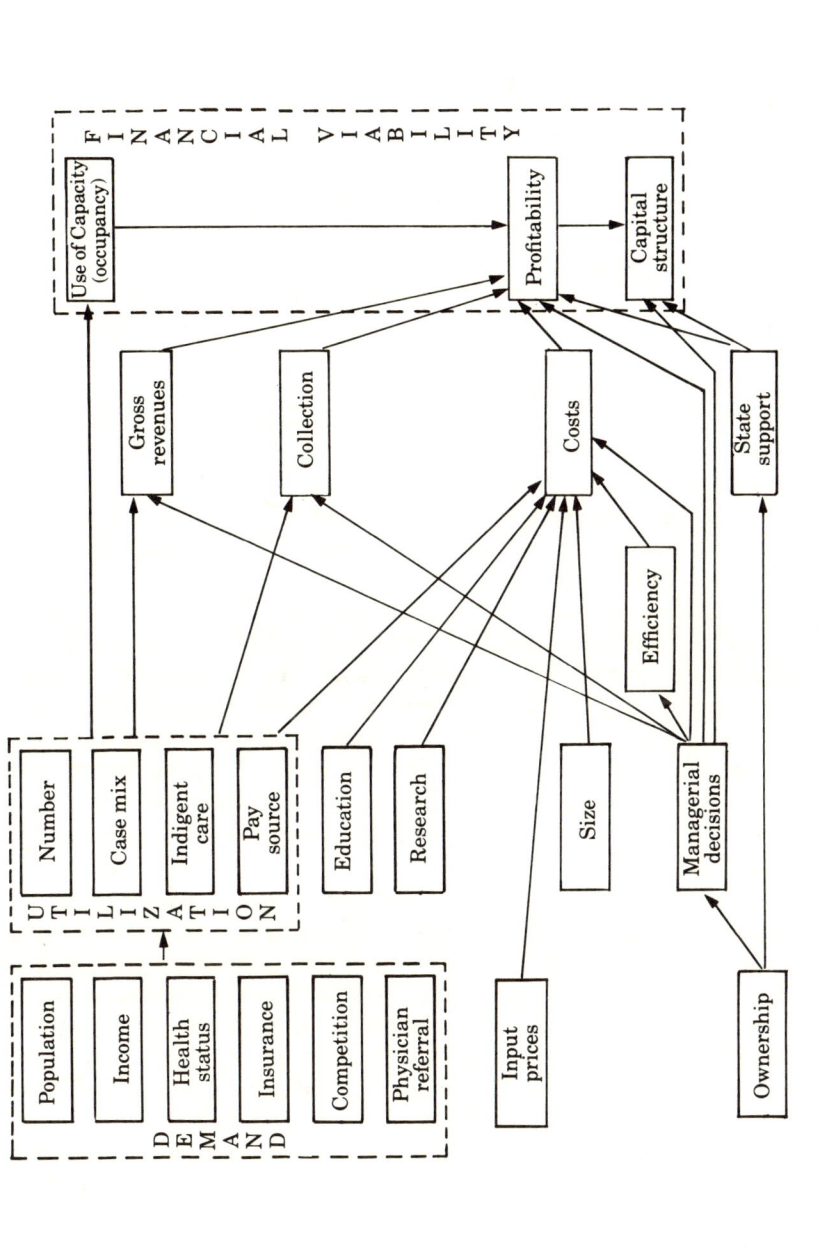

Figure 8.1 Model of University Hospital Financial Viability

total costs will increase with size, but the theoretical relationship between size and cost per admission, or average cost, has been suggested to be U-shaped; that is, costs per admission will decrease with increased size until a certain point is reached when diseconomies of scale will come into effect and cause costs per admission to increase. However, as university hospitals are medium to large size, the observed relationship between size and costs is likely to be on the second half of the U-shaped curve, that is, on the positive slope. This suggests that university hospital costs per admission will increase with size.

The remaining major determinant of costs is hypothesized to be the nature of managerial decisions within the university hospital—both directly regarding the level and nature of services as well as alternative inputs, and indirectly through the level of efficiency of those inputs, chiefly labor and supplies.

The level and nature of managerial decisions in university-owned hospitals will be determined by the unique ownership and governance structure. Whether the hospital belongs to a public or private university will influence the governance structure and management autonomy to some degree. Furthermore, ownership will also affect the level of state support (financial and otherwise).

We hypothesized that state support has a direct effect upon the profitability of the public hospital and a direct effect on its capital structure. Greater state appropriations reduce the need to go to the debt market to raise money for capital replacement.

The other major factors affecting capital structure are managerial decisions such as choosing between going into debt or raising funds in other ways for capital improvements or replacement, or whether the hospital's profits (excess over expenses) necessitate incurring debt to raise funds for such projects.

As figure 8.1 shows, the profitability of a university hospital is hypothetically determined by all of the characteristics except capital structure. We have not yet discussed gross revenues and its related factor, collection. Both are an integral part of the level of profitability. Gross patient revenues can be thought of as a function of the number of services provided and the prices charged for those services. However, not all payers pay the full price, and some payers reimburse on the basis of costs, not charges. Thus, the collection rate reflects the proportion of gross revenues received after contractual, bad debt, and charity allowances have been subtracted. This collection rate will depend on the type of patients admitted and their method of payment for services. For example, the higher the level of indigent care, the higher will be the charity allowance and the bad debt allowance. Contractual allowances will be higher when more patients are covered by the cost-based third-party payers. Of course both the gross patient revenues and the collection rate will be affected by managerial decisions, which determine the prices charged for services and the efforts made to reduce the level of deductions and collect unpaid accounts.

The level of profitability is the most important component of financial viability. A university hospital must be able to earn an excess of revenues over expenses in the long run in order to survive. The profitability measure being used in this study, operating margin (OPMAR), includes any state appropriations received by university-owned hospitals. This approach recognizes the importance of state support in assessing financial viability. The second most important component of financial viability is the hospital's capital structure, measured here as the ratio of long-term debt to net fixed assets (LTDNFA). Hospitals with relatively low rates of debt financing are more likely to be able to borrow money—both to finance replacement and expansion, and to finance short-term losses. We hypothesized that use of capacity, as represented by occupancy (OCC), is important but somewhat less so than OPMAR and LTDNFA. A hospital with high occupancy is using its resources efficiently, and one with low occupancy has resources available not being put to use. However, neither of these conditions guarantees good or bad financial performance; they are merely contributing factors.

Finally, the level of profitability will also be affected by hospital capacity, which is in turn a direct result of the utilization of the hospital.

METHODOLOGY AND MEASURES

Measures of Financial Viability

The data for this part of the study were obtained from the responses of 52 university-owned teaching hospitals to the *Council on Teaching Hospitals' Survey of Financial and General Operating Data* for the fiscal year ending in 1981, and from the 1982 management and governance survey sponsored by the Consortium for the Study of University Hospitals [12].

Although the COTH survey concentrates on income statement information, there were enough items on the questionnaire to provide a picture of the hospital's financial position. The specific measures used to capture the concept of financial viability were: (1) the operating margin ratio (total operating revenue minus operating expenses, divided by total operating revenue), used to measure profitability; (2) the ratio of long-term debt to net fixed assets, used as a measure of capital structure; and (3) the percent of occupancy (patient days/bed days available) as a measure of the use of capacity. These variables are shown in table 8.1.

Of the hospitals studied, 17 have negative operating margins, while the most common margin is between 3 and 4 percent. Most hospitals use very little long-term debt, so that their ratios of long-term debt to net fixed assets (LTDNFA) are very low. Thirteen fall in a group with LTDNFA from .20 to .45 while 10 hospitals have a ratio of more than .5. The mean occupancy of these university-owned hospitals is 79 percent, with 8 hospitals experiencing occupancy rates of less than 72 percent.

Obviously, the hospitals with the highest level of financial viability, that is, the greatest chance of survival, are those with high occupancy, a high operating margin, and a low level of net fixed assets financed by long-term debt. However, there is the problem of how to distinguish good viability from poor viability when one or two ratios are high and the others low.

Given the earlier assumptions about the relative importance of OPMAR, LTDNFA, and OCC, we developed a composite continuous measure of financial viability for each hospital by standardizing their values (i.e., with a mean of zero and standard deviation equal to one). That is, we summed these values, giving the operating margin a weighting of 2, LTDFNA a weighting of 1, and occupancy a weighting of 0.5. The weightings are somewhat arbitrary, but the intention was to reflect the relative importance of the components of the composite measure. (LTDFNA was converted by subtracting its value from one in order to represent the proportion of net fixed assets not financed by long term debt, so that "higher" would mean "better," and thus be

Table 8.1 Component Variables of Financial Viability

Variable	N	Minimum Value	Maximum Value	Mean	Standard Deviation
Operating margin (OPMAR) (profitability)	48	−0.2203	0.1160	0.0087	0.0663
Long term debt to net fixed assets (LTDNFA) (capital structure)	51	0.000	1.3646	0.2623	0.3374
Occupancy (OCC) (use of capacity)	52	63.0000	93.0000	79.0800	6.4500

consistent with the other variables.) The higher the measure, the greater the financial viability.

The result of this composite score gave a measure of financial viability ranging from −8.14 to 3.94, with 21 hospitals having values less than 0 and 26 hospitals with measures greater than 0.

Operationalization of Independent Variables

Most of the factors hypothesized to influence financial viability (figure 8.1) have been included in the empirical analysis to follow. These factors are represented by the measures described in table 8.2. Additional comments about some of these measures follow below.

The level of competition (*COMP*) facing the university hospital was measured by the responses of the Chief Executive Officers to the CSUH survey question, "How many of the hospitals in your primary service area would you consider to be competitive with yours?"

Medical staff characteristics (*STAFF*) were measured by the response to a question on the CSUH survey, "What proportion of your active physicians have affiliations with other hospitals?" Five possible answers were given: (i) 0 percent coded as 1; (ii) 1–25 percent coded as 2; (iii) 26–50 percent coded as 3; (iv) 51–75 percent coded as 4; and (v) 76+ percent coded as 5. While this measure does not capture the full range of medical staff characteristics (such as specialty, teaching, and research involvement), it does provide a valuable indication of the location of privileges and physicians' likelihood of admitting patients to the university hospital.

Wages (*WAGE*) were measured by the payroll expenses per full-time employee as computed from the results of the American Hospital Association's *Annual Survey of Hospitals, 1980* [13]. While a more extensive hospital wage index would have been preferred, this measure does represent the differences in salaries between hospitals in different locations, assuming that each hospital has approximately the same proportion of employees at each level.

Ownership (*OWN*) was represented by a categorical variable, where 1 = public university ownership and 2 = private university ownership.

The number of patients (*ADM*) was represented by the number of admissions to each university hospital as reported on the COTH survey of 1981. The inclusion of outpatient visits might have provided a more complete picture of the number of patients, but this was assumed to be in proportion to the number of admissions and thus would not change the relative levels of different hospitals.

Case mix (*MIX*) was a complex variable to measure, but for pur-

Table 8.2 Description of Independent Variables

Abbreviation	Variable	Mean	Standard Deviation
POP	Population in state in 1980	8,015,550	6,549,400
INC	Per capita income of state ($)	8,663	1,040
COMP	Number of competitors	4.45	4.15
STAFF	Proportion of physicians with other affiliations	2.39	1.19
WAGE	Payroll expenses per employee ($)	14,001	2,985
OWN	Ownership	1.35	0.23
ADM	Admissions	18,024	5,293
MIX	Tertiarity	2.77	0.43
INDIG	Degree of indigent care	1.76	0.74
PAY	Percent of revenues from government	57.2	15.0
EDUC	House staff per bed	0.44	0.16
BEDS	Beds	545	171
CAPFIN	Managerial influence over capital decisions	0.19	0.10
OPBUD	Managerial influence over operating budget	0.29	0.13
GOVORG	Managerial influence over organization and governance	0.13	0.07
EFF	Employees per bed	4.77	1.16
GRREV	Gross patient revenues per admission ($)	5,457	1,289
REVDED	Revenue deduction rate (%)	0.19	0.11
COST	Expenses per admission ($)	4,669	1,188
STATE	State appropriation per admission ($)	361	554

poses of simplicity was represented by the response to a CSUH question regarding the perception of the hospital as a site for highly specialized care. To the extent that these perceptions are valid, this measures tertiary care.

The level of indigent care (*INDIG*) was measured by the response to a question about the extent to which the community perceived the hospital to be a place for indigent care. This variable is also dependent on the validity of the perceptions.

The type of pay source (*PAY*) of patients seen at each university hospital was represented by the percentage of net patient revenues received from government sources as opposed to private sources such as commercial insurance, Blue Cross and self-paying patients. We chose this variable to indicate the level of reimbursement given to each hospital, as private sources are more likely to reimburse at a level close to gross revenues or charges.

We measured the level of education (*EDUC*) by the number of house staff per bed as computed from results of the COTH survey. We considered an alternative measure—the value of educational costs per bed. However, the former measure seemed to be more appropriate in differentiating between levels of educational activity without confounding the measure with cost differences.

Size (*BEDS*) was measured by the number of beds in each hospital in 1981 as reported on the COTH survey.

Using the responses from the CSUH survey, we translated the level of managerial decisions in university hospitals into measures. These measures describe the level of influence that hospital administration has in three type of decisions: the amount and source of capital financing (*CAPFIN*), operating budget decisions (*OPBUD*), and reorganization at the governance level that gave substantial autonomy to the university hospital (*GOVORG*). For all three variables, the higher value means that the hospital administration has greater influence.

We measured efficiency (*EFF*) by using COTH's survey data to compute the number of full-time employees per bed. This variable can be interpreted as a measure of efficiency or productivity, where low values are favorable. Another interpretation sees the variable as a measure of quality, where increased values represent potential improvements in the quality of care. However, the former interpretation seems to us to be more appropriate; all other things being equal (such as quality and level of service produced), fewer employees mean increased productivity.

Gross patient revenues (*GRREV*) were measured by the value of gross patient revenues per admission, computed from the COTH data. By using a per-unit approach, the measure can be standardized for size and level of utilization.

Revenue deduction rate (*REVDED*) was captured by a ratio of gross patient revenues minus net patient revenues, divided by gross patient revenues, again calculated from data reported to COTH. This measures the extent to which net patient revenues differ from what was actually charged.

Costs (*COST*) were measured by COTH data calculated to create an expression of the total expenses per admission to the hospital. As with the revenue concept, this was standardized per unit of admission.

State support (*STATE*) was measured by the amount of state appropriations per admission, as reported in the COTH study.

RESULTS

The conceptual model specified earlier (see figure 8.1) was tested using path analysis. This type of analysis amounts to a series of multiple regressions and allows the disaggregation of total observed effects of the university hospital characteristics (the independent variables described in table 8.2) into (1) direct effects, (2) indirect effects through all the paths between the characteristics and financial viability, the dependent variable (viability), and (3) effects due to common correlation with other preceding characteristics in the model. The model was tested by determining the significance of the path coefficients. Those path coefficients that were significant represented valid parts of the model. The path coefficients were calculated by multiple-regression analyses performed on the standardized variables, thus giving standardized partial regression coefficients. This form of regression provides information concerning the relative importance of the different independent variables in predicting the dependent variable. Furthermore, the standardization of the coefficients allows us to compute products of coefficients to determine the size of the indirect effects of the characteristics upon viability. The square of the multiple correlation coefficient, R^2, provided the amount of variation in a variable that could be explained by those characteristics preceding it.

The results of the path analysis are indicated in figure 8.2, with financial viability expressed as a single composite measure. Only those characteristics with statistically significant path coefficients (at the .10 level) are included. The equation for financial viability explains 63 percent of its variation, indicating that the model was reasonably well-formulated.

Figure 8.3 shows the statistically significant path coefficients and their explanation of the variation in occupancy (OCC), operating margin (OPMARG), and long-term debt to net fixed assets (LTDNFA). The equations for occupancy, operating margin, and long-term debt to net fixed assets explained 28, 64, and 24 percent of their respective variations.

Comparison of figures 8.1, 8.2 and 8.3 indicates that gross revenues, collection rates and costs are significantly related to financial viability through their impact on hospitals' operating margins, as predicted. However, the influence of state support was somewhat surprising. Although increased state support is associated with reduced long-term debt ratios, and to a much lesser extent with improved operating margins, its impact on the overall concept of financial viability as specifically defined for this chapter is not significant. The obvious relationship between public university ownership and higher levels of state support was substantiated by the analysis.

The model provided an explanation of 77 percent of the variation in university hospitals' costs. The characteristics with significant path coefficients contributing to costs are hospital size, number of admissions, efficiency (employees per bed), input prices and the level of indigent care. Increases in any of these variables are related to increased costs per admission with the exception of the number of admissions. Increased admissions are associated with reduced costs. Notably missing in this explanation of university hospitals were our hypothesized effects of the level of educational activity, managerial decisions, and the level of tertiary care.

On the revenue side, the model is less useful, providing equations that explain only 19 percent of the variations in both gross revenues per admission and the collection rate (the difference between gross revenues and net revenues). The level of indigent care is the only variable related to the collection rate. In fact, increased levels of indigent care are associated with smaller differences between gross and net revenues, indicating that those hospitals providing more indigent care have fewer deductions from gross revenue. Surprisingly (though consistent with findings reported in earlier chapters), hospitals in states with higher levels of per capita income are likely to provide more indigent care.

Increased gross patient revenues are associated with greater managerial influence of the operating budget, less managerial influence over capital financing, and a higher percent of patients with government payment sources.

The size of the population in the state where each university hospital is located is significantly related to the percentage of hospital business coming from the government. University hospitals in more heavily populated states are likely to have more government-paying patients, and to have a higher level of tertiary care.

The variable describing the level of tertiary care is directly and positively related to financial viability. Other variables having a direct effect on viability, as predicted, are the three managerial influence variables in the areas of operational budgeting, governance reorganization, and capital financing. Increased influence over the first two areas are related to improved viability, but increased managerial influ-

Figure 8.2 Results of Path Analysis for a Single Measure of Viability

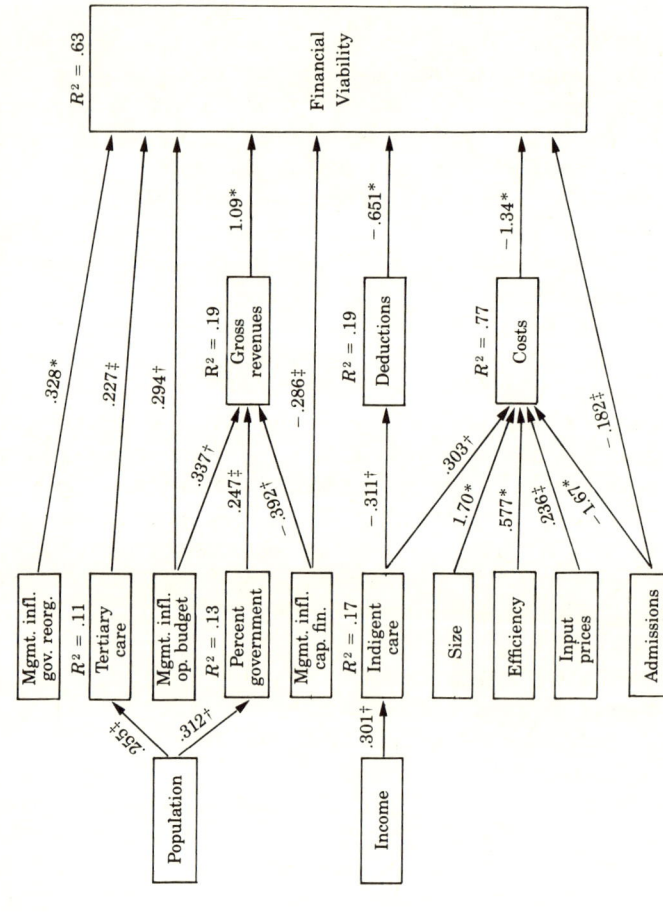

Note: Unstandardized path coefficients used here.
*$p \leq .01$.
†$p \leq .05$.
‡$p \leq .10$.

Figure 8.3 Results of Path Analysis for Three Viability Measures

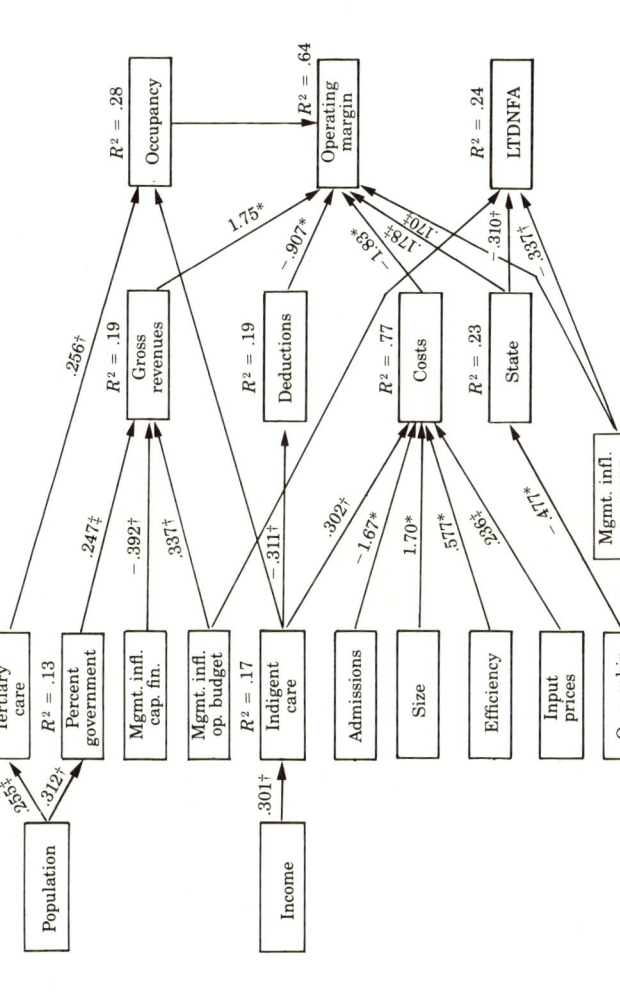

Note: Unstandardized path coefficients used here.
*$p \leq .01$.
†$p \leq .05$.
‡$p \leq .10$.

132 / *Governing University Hospitals*

ence over capital financing is associated with reduced financial viability for university hospitals.

Examination of figure 8.3 shows the nature of the effects of managerial decisions on the components of financial viability. Reduced levels of long-term debt are associated with increased managerial influence over operational budgeting and governance reorganization, but not with the level of managerial influence over capital financing decisions. In addition, the results shown in figure 8.3 indicate that the relationship between tertiary care and the use of capacity (or occupancy) does exist as hypothesized. Contrary to the hypotheses presented in figure 8.1, neither the level of competition in the university hospitals' primary service areas nor the percentage of medical staff affiliated with other hospitals are significantly related to any of the utilization components (e.g., admissions, level of tertiary and indigent care, and type of patient pay source). Furthermore, the hypothesized effect of the type of ownership on the extent of managerial influence is not supported by the analysis.

So far we have described the direct effects of university hospital characteristics on both financial viability and other characteristics. Now we use the path analysis to examine both the direct and indirect effects of variables hypothesized to influence financial viability. Earlier, we hypothesized that utilization would influence financial viability both directly and indirectly through its effects on revenues and costs. Figure 8.2 shows that to some extent these hypothesized relationships are supported by the data. A higher number of admissions has a small and negative direct effect on financial viability. However, admissions have a large positive indirect effect on financial viability because admissions were associated with reduced costs, and reduced costs are associated with increased viability. The magnitude of this indirect effect through costs is equal to the product of the coefficient of admissions on costs and the coefficient of costs on financial viability, or

$$(-1.6651) \times (-1.3446) = 2.23889.$$

This indirect effect of admissions on financial viability is far greater than its direct effect, which equals only $-.18197$. The overall effects of admissions on financial viability thus equals the sum of the direct and indirect effects, or

$$(-.18197) + (2.23889) = 2.05692.$$

Hence, other things being equal, higher admissions result in better financial performance.

Another important characteristic to evaluate in this manner is hospital size, which is not directly related to viability but has a strong negative relationship with viability because bed size is associated with higher average costs. Therefore, both fewer beds and more admissions are associated with improved financial performance. Two viability-enhancing strategies are suggested by these results. First, university hospitals should determine whether they can increase admissions through expanded market share. Second, those who cannot should move promptly to reduce the size of their acute care operation.

Other characteristics positively related to viability are the level of managerial influence over reorganization and operational budgeting, percentage of government patients, level of tertiary care, and to a lesser extent population size and per capita income. Still other characteristics negatively related to viability are increased numbers of employees per bed (i.e., decreased efficiency), increased managerial influence over capital financing, and higher levels of indigent care.

EFFECTS OF UNIVERSITY HOSPITAL OWNERSHIP

Differences between private and state-owned university hospitals deserve special note. Of the study hospitals, 34 are owned by state universities and 18 by private universities. Ideally we would have analyzed each group separately, but the small number of private hospitals prevented this. However, exploratory correlational analysis indicates that ownership does indeed affect the way in which university hospital characteristics affect viability.

Ownership is associated with both the level of occupancy and the ratio of long-term debt to net fixed assets. In general, private university-owned hospitals experienced higher levels of occupancy during 1981 than those owned by state universities. As might have been predicted, private university hospitals had higher levels of debt, largely because they do not receive as much state financial support—thus necessitating greater use of the debt market for raising capital.

One striking area where ownership makes a difference is the level of managerial influence over decision making. The viability of private university-owned hospitals is strongly related to the variables representing the level of managerial influence over capital financing, operational budgeting, and governance reorganization decisions. The viability of state university-owned hospitals is not strongly related to these variables.

CONCLUSIONS

This study has identified certain characteristics of university hospitals that are related to the financial viability of university hospitals. Principal among these characteristics are the level of gross revenues, the collection rate, and the level of costs. In addition, while state support is not related to the viability of private university hospitals, for public university hospitals the level of state support is an important determinant of viability. This analysis has provided some understanding of the determinants of university hospital costs, but it has been less successful in explaining the level of gross revenues and net revenues. Further investigation in this area is necessary to provide information concerning ways to increase university hospital revenues.

University hospitals should examine closely their pricing structures, as the level of revenues they receive is so crucial to their viability. They should seek additional sources of revenue to cover all of their activities. According to our 1981 data, current sources of revenue such as Medicaid and Medicare do not appear to be adversely affecting financial viability and operating margins. However, since then, considerable changes have occurred in Medicaid and Medicare payment; a study of 1984 data might indicate more government, Medicaid, or Medicare payments are less favorable in determining financial viability.

In university hospitals costs are associated with utilization and input prices in the same way as in community hospitals, and they are a crucial element of financial viability. Although increased indigent care was associated with better collection rates (less difference between gross and net revenues), the overall impact on viability was negative, because more indigent care increased costs. Governing bodies of university hospitals should be made aware of the inherent difficulties involved in providing costly indigent care while trying to maintain centers of excellence and leadership in health care education and research. If this role as indigent care providers is to continue, university hospitals must be compensated appropriately for their costs.

We also found that larger size was a fundamental characteristic of university hospitals experiencing viability problems. University hospitals might have to become even more specialized and concentrate totally on tertiary care in order to reduce their size to manageable levels. Alternatively, university hospitals could be operated as several distinct units to increase manageability and reduce the inherent size problem. Ironically, perhaps the size of the institution allows more complex tertiary care to be performed, thus creating higher costs and reduced viability. Further studies should include a far more precise measure of the type of care provided and examine its relationship with size and costs.

One fundamental element of university hospitals does not appear to be associated with viability: the level of educational involvement. Because of their contribution to costs, educational activities should be monitored carefully. However, our study does not indicate that university hospitals should change this part of their mission in order to remain viable.

Finally, the level of managerial influence or autonomy, while not apparently related to the control of costs, does seem to be associated with improved financial viability.

REFERENCES

1. Wayne, M.E., and R. Plakowski. Educational costs to hospitalized patients. *Journal of Medical Education* 53(1978):383–86.
2. Schroeder, S.A., and D.S. O'Leary. Differences in laboratory use and length of stay between university and community hospitals. *Journal of Medical Education* 52(1977):418–20.
3. Worthington, N.L. The effects of graduate medical education upon hospital utilization and costs. Paper presented at the American Public Health Association meetings, November 1982.
4. Sloan, F.A., R.D. Feldman, and B. Steinwald. Effects of teaching on hospital costs. *Journal of Health Economics* 2(1983):1–28.
5. Ament, R.P., E.J. Kobrinski, and W.R. Wood. Case mix competing between teaching and nonteaching hospitals. *Journal of Medical Education* 56(1981):894–903.
6. Busby, D.D., J.C. Leming, and M.I. Olson. Unidentified educational costs in a university teaching hospital: An initial study. *Journal of Medical Education* 47(1972):243–53.
7. Isaacs, J. Net patient revenue at university-owned teaching hospitals. *Journal of Medical Education* 57(1982):731–33.
8. ———. Analysis of university-owned teaching hospitals' income. *Journal of Medical Education* 56(1981):783–85.
9. Penchansky, R., and B. Steinhauer. The specialty referral centers: Prospects and consequences. University of Michigan, unpublished, 1982.
10. Westerman, J.H. A requiem for the university hospital? *Health Care Management Review* 5(Spring 1980):17–24.
11. Schramm, C.J. The teaching hospital and the future role of state government. *New England Journal of Medicine* 308(1983):41–45.
12. Isaacs, J. *COTH survey of university-owned teaching hospitals' financial and general operating data. 1981.* Washington, D.C.: Department of Teaching Hospitals, Association of American Medical Colleges, 1983.
13. American Hospital Association. *Annual Survey of Hospitals, 1980.* Chicago: American Hospital Association.

NINE

Managing Support Services in University Hospitals

The earlier chapters have examined the effect of various factors on the university hospital as a whole, now we focus our perspective on a crucial part of the hospital enterprise: support services—that broad and varied group of hospital activities necessary to support the medical enterprise. This chapter addresses the issue of managing support services in university hospitals, and the factors that make the managing of these services so difficult.

A major concern of many university hospital administrators is their lack of control over these services. The data in our study have confirmed that in many of these hospitals control is in fact at other levels in the academic health center (AHC), the university, or the state. However, the study results give only weak support to a relationship between control of support services and hospital performance, and we draw instead from the experience of several field-study hospitals to suggest that responsiveness of support services to hospital needs may be achieved by means other than controlling them at the hospital level.

The main problem in managing hospital support services is that many of those services are directly paralleled in other parts of the academic health center, the university, or the state. These other levels may have an interest in controlling such services in the hospital as well. For example, the university can centralize the hospital's purchasing, personnel, and general accounting by managing the policy and procedure control directly. Hospital administrators may thus have limited authority in these areas, yet be held responsible by their hospital colleagues for the effectiveness of these support services. University hospital administrators who are forced to share control with groups in the ownership environment, or accept total control from them, have a vivid understanding of the difficulties this creates [1,2]. These services are really the basic "if-you-can't-handle-this-nothing-else-matters" issue for hospital administration. It is not the most important set of problems facing them, but there is a sense that if hospital administration cannot keep the floor clean and the units staffed, there is something wrong with hospital administration.

DATA SOURCES AND SCORING

The data on support services control come from the survey (see chapter 2, table 3) completed in each study hospital by a member of the administrative staff, who showed the reporting line and the source and degree of external policy control for each of 20 support services. From this data, we quantified the concept of control over a support service by measuring the extent of direct supervisory responsibility for a service, and the extent of policy and procedure control. Because policy and procedure control (e.g., the state specifying policy and procedures for hiring, discipline, or pay scales) has less direct impact, it was given less weight than direct supervisory control. The following weights were assigned:

Exclusive supervisory control	= 1.00
Shared supervisory control	= 0.50
Nonsupervisory policy and procedure control	= 0.66
Nonsupervisory general policy guidance	= 0.33

We calculated control scores for each decision-making group that had some control over the 20 support services. For example, if in one hospital the hospital administration had exclusive supervisory control over all 20 services, the "HA" score was 20 (20 × 1.0). If for 12 services the university laid down specific rules and procedures, the "university" score was 8 (0.66 × 12). If for 6 services the state provided general guidelines, the "state" score was 2 (0.33 × 6). We also calculated control scores by service, adding the control scores of each group for that service.

To test for the influence of support service control on the performance of the hospital, we developed four measures of "efficiency in resource utilization" from 1981 financial and operating data submitted annually to the Council of Teaching Hospitals (COTH) of the Association of American Medical Colleges (AAMC)[3]. We reversed scales where necessary so that a high score reflected high efficiency. The four efficiency scales are:

1. *Number of personnel per adjusted bed* (reversed), a statistic that shows the number of full-time equivalent personnel (FTEs) per bed. This figure is adjusted for outpatient services, based on the ratio of dollar volume in outpatient services to the dollar volume in inpatient services.
2. *Inventory per occupied bed* (reversed), a statistic that divides year-end inventory by the average number of occupied beds during the year.
3. *Average days in receivables* (reversed), a statistic that divides average daily revenues by average receivables outstanding.
4. *Growth-adjusted occupancy,* a statistic that adjusts average daily occupancy upward (downward) in proportion with occupancy increases (decreases) in two prior years.

FINDINGS

There is substantial variation among support services in the degree to which they are externally controlled. Table 9.1 orders the support services according to the degree they are controlled by hospital administration.

It is evident that patient-related support services (pharmacy, social service, admitting) appear at the top of the list, and are followed by the administrative support services that might appear in any large organization. This order appears to be a function of medical-professional control and also of the degree to which the service is unique to the hospital (not present in other parts of the university). Although the table provides a relatively accurate picture of formal control, it does not show the degree to which services controlled by groups outside the hospital are responsive to the hospital's needs. The absence of formal control by the hospital need not mean a lack of responsiveness of the support service to hospital needs, though it does make that responsiveness more problematic.

A hospital-by-hospital analysis of these 20 support services shows a wide distribution of control, shown in table 9.2. It is evident from the

Table 9.1 Degree of Hospital Control of Support Services

Support Services	Hospital Supervisory Control of Service (Range: 0–15)
Pharmacy	15.0
Social services	15.0
Admitting	15.0
Patient accounting	14.5
Volunteers	14.5
Food services	13.5
Housekeeping	13.5
Laundry/linen	12.5
Data processing	11.0
Engineering/methods	11.0
Material management/stores	9.5
General accounting	8.5
Payroll	8.0
Personnel	7.0
Security	6.5
Maintenance	6.0
Public relations/fund raising	5.5
Purchasing	4.5
Renovation/plant engineering	4.5
Parking	1.0

table that in two hospitals (numbers 14 and 15), the academic health center (AHC) and University have more control over support services than does the hospital administration. In another half-dozen (8 through 13), there is little difference between the two columns.

The table does not show the state as having major control over support services in any of the study hospitals, but this is misleading for the presence of control at higher levels has been shown to increase formalization of procedures and encourages centralized controls [4]. State influence is common in purchasing, personnel, and general accounting, three areas that can be formalized and centralized at the university level. Most hospital administrators feel constrained by this control. However, in one of the study hospitals, the hospital administrator felt that the real constraint is the margin of safety the university administrators add to ensure compliance with the state control.

Our first question is, "What is the degree of association between hospital control of support services and performance?" The correlation between control and the four measures of hospital efficiency is shown in the first column of table 9.3. A positive relationship between hospital control and efficiency is given some support: the higher the control

Table 9.2 Distribution of Control of Support Services

Hospital	Control by Hospital (Max Score = 20)	Control by AHC or University (Max Score = 20)	Control by State (Max Score = 20)	Total Control Score
1	19.5	.5	0	20.0
2	18.5	1.8	4.0	24.3
3	18.0	4.3	.5	22.8
4	17.0	6.3	0	23.3
5	14.5	5.5	0	20.0
6	14.5	7.0	3.5	25.0
7	14.0	8.3	0	22.3
8	11.5	8.5	0	20.0
9	11.5	9.5	0	21.0
10	11.5	9.7	2.5	23.7
11	11.5	10.8	2.5	24.8
12	11.0	11.7	1.5	24.2
13	10.0	10.0	0	20.0
14	7.5	12.0	4.0	23.5
15	5.5	14.5	2.0	22.0

Note: Basis for control scores:
1.0 = Exclusive control;
0.5 = Shared control;
0.66 = Provides specific rules, forms, procedures;
0.33 = Provides general policy guidance.

by hospital administration, the higher the efficiency. Three of the four correlations are in the expected direction, and one reaches statistical significance.

The relationship is somewhat strengthened when AHC control is added to hospital administration control (table 9.3, second column). The one exception is in growth-adjusted occupancy, perhaps the least sensitive of the four to effective management of support services. The favorable effect of AHC influence is an important finding; it gives support to the possibility that if support services are responsive to hospital requirements, control need not reside at the hospital level. The expected negative relation between state or university level and efficiency is also given some support (see table 9.3, third column). Three of the four correlations are in the expected negative direction and one reaches statistical significance.

Our next question is, "What is the association between multiple control over support services and hospital efficiency?" We reviewed data for the six key support services most often identified in our inter-

Table 9.3 Relation of Support Service Control with Hospital Efficiency Indicators,* Rank Correlations ($N = 14$)

	Hospital Administration Control with:	HA and Academic Health Center Control with:	State and University Control with:
Number of personnel per adjusted bed†	.23	.34	−.10
Inventory per occupied bed	.49	.55	−.05
Average days in receivables	−.18	.22	−.56
Growth-adjusted occupancy‡	.23	−.01	+.06

*All data for fiscal year ending in 1981.
†"Adjusted bed" is a statistic that increases the number of beds in proportion to the dollar volume of outpatient services.
‡"Growth adjusted occupancy" adjusts actual occupancy upward (downward) in proportion to occupancy increases (decreases) in two prior years.

views as a source of difficulty (data processing, general accounting, payroll, personnel, maintenance, and purchasing) in order to determine the extent of multiple supervisory and policy control. We then calculated multiple control scores for each hospital. The results are shown in table 9.4.

The one exception, "average days in receivables," is a positive correlation. The predominant relationship between multiple control of support services and efficiency is negative, giving some support to the proposition that "too many cooks spoil the broth." Clarity of support service control—as well as its location—appears to influence performance.

DISCUSSION

The findings on the one hand give some support to a position widely held by university hospital administrators, that they are less economically efficient if they are denied the right to manage their own support services. On the other hand the support for this position is weak, and suggests that control of support services at higher levels of the organization may have some counterjustification. At least four reasons can explain why organizations at a higher level seek to control the operation of services at some lower organization level.

Table 9.4 Relationship of Multiple Control over Support Services with Hospital Efficiency Indicators, Rank Correlations ($N = 14$)

	Multiple Control with
Number of personnel per adjusted bed	−.18
Inventory per occupied bed	−.45
Average days in receivables	+.30
Growth adjusted occupancy	−.23

1. *Economies of scale.* Purchasing is a common example, and a valid one. Indeed, many hospitals in the United States have set up or participate in joint purchasing arrangements [5]. The difficulty for university hospitals is that in many cases they are obtaining fewer economies by joint purchasing with other parts of the university or state than they would obtain with other hospitals. Security or maintenance are perhaps better examples of support services that can achieve economies of scale when operated at the university level. It is difficult to find appropriate economies of scale at the state level.

2. *Interdependence among units.* Personnel policies are a good illustration of interdependence between the hospital and other university units. Inconsistent salary, benefits, or vacation policies can indeed be a major irritant to good personnel relations when they occur among people who work closely together. But uniformity also has its costs [6]. In one of the field-study hospitals, hiring was frozen because the university had a surplus of clerks. The timing of this freeze worked against hospital needs. The point of view of the university was understandable; they wanted to place their surplus clericals in the hospital if the occasion arose. However, the hospital was faced with the prospect of extensive retraining of unqualified personnel. Hiring competent personnel would have been more cost efficient and effective. Interdependence is also clearly illustrated in fund raising, public relations, and state relations. In state relations, for example, it is obviously important that a state university and its hospital coordinate closely in appropriation requests.

3. *Low managerial competence in the hospital.* University hospi-

tals are not widely used as examples of excellence in management, and we heard several "horror stories" in which university officials took control of an activity that was being managed poorly by the hospital. There is a solid logic for having appropriate monitoring of the performance of university hospitals, or even the temporary provision of services when these cannot be managed well. However when neither scale economies nor interdependence justifies centralized control of a support service, it may be wiser to deal with low managerial competence by improving the hospital's management, rather than by centralizing the function. University hospitals are too complex, and operate in too dynamic an environment, to survive without good management [7]. Low managerial competence is a reason for changes in the management of hospitals. It is unlikely that a shift of that responsibility upward to the university or state will be a successful solution.

4. *Preservation of traditional practices.* The structures of decision making and control in state and university bureaucracies tend to persist, independent of the reasons that originally gave rise to them [8]. Practices that have given power and discretion to key figures in the university and state will be defended by those who derive their power from them. Every university will have functionally organized units responsible for monitoring and sometimes directly providing support services. Often headed by able and influential vice-presidents, these departments are accustomed to providing a broad range of services that often include the whole lower end of the support services list. They are, moreover, accustomed to providing these services to academic departments, known for their low interest in the operation of such services. The heads of the functional departments are thus conditioned to expect they will play an important role guiding "their" function, and the hospital is seen by them as part of their domain. Persons who have moved that far up the university hierarchy will not wish to lose their influence, and thus the simple politics of power will be an important reason for retaining control of support services at the university level. The same dynamic, with different actors, operates at the state level.

University hospital administrators do not object to securing economies of scale or to structures that deal effectively with interdependence. (University control of parking, for example, is almost universally supported.) Their objections focus much more on supervisory control of support services at the university or state level because "We can do it better" (managerial competence argument) or because "It's always been that way" (the traditional practices argument). In one of the hospitals we visited, receivables had risen rapidly over a several-month period because a modernizing of the patient accounts system had so confused the accounts that the hospital was unable to get any patient bills out for three months. (Under these circumstances, receivables rise very rapidly indeed!) However, this decision was not made at the hospital. It started at the hospital, went up to the next level, went from there up to university administration, and the final decision was really diffused over several levels. There was, we have to say, managerial incompetence, but it was not all at the hospital level. The issue is not whether patient accounts receivables should be well managed; of course they should be. The issue is where an action that may include decisions about data processing, capital budget allocations, personnel policies, and patient accounts receivables can be made expeditiously and without diffusing responsibility for results to such a degree that no one is responsible.

In another university hospital, our field-study visit coincided with a great victory over the state civil service by the hospital; a year of sustained effort by the hospital administrator and his chief financial officer had finally secured them the right to pay the university hospital personnel officer a salary that would allow them to recruit and retain the quality of person they believed was necessary. But these are costly battles to wage.

As environments grow more complex and the core technologies of hospitals become more sharply differentiated from other parts of the university or state, there is a growing need for support services such as personnel, purchasing, or data processing to be responsive to hospital needs [9]. Control at higher levels than the hospital means that the administrative matters associated with coordinating support services cannot be delegated, but must be dealt with at the top of the hospital's administrative structure. First-rate administrators do not tolerate that well. Either they leave, or cease to be first-rate administrators. As one said on turning down an offer to move to a much larger university hospital, "If I were going to move now, I'd move to a private."

METHODS OF SECURING RESPONSIVE SUPPORT SERVICES

Although some of the reasons for control of hospital support services by the AHC, university, or state are not persuasive, certainly the potential for economies of scale and the presence of interdependence are quite valid reasons. The presence of such factors may help explain why hospital efficiency indicators are not more closely related to hospital control of support services. The correlational data reported earlier leave room for the possibility that the responsiveness of support services is the key variable, and having exclusive control over them is only one way the hospital has of achieving that responsiveness. From the experience of the 15 study hospitals, we can identify three rather different solutions that are used with some success to manage the support service problem set.

The first solution is, of course, hospital control of these services. This solution is well exemplified by Johns Hopkins Hospital or Shands Teaching Hospital at the University of Florida, which accept almost total responsibility for the operation of these services. Both of these hospitals have the legal form of a separate corporation. Hopkins is, in fact, quite separate from Johns Hopkins University in history, in board composition, and in the locus of decision-making power. Thus, at Hopkins the hospital control of support services is simply a by-product of separate ownership. At Florida the need for hospital control of support services was a major reason to incorporate separately, for the state control of university services was hindering the effective performance of these services in the hospital. Key groups in the legislature, the governor's office, the university administration, and the medical school all agreed on a structure that would make Shands Hospital legally separate from the university, and therefore from state control. This is the model that many university hospital administrators see as the ideal.

A second solution is the AHC model, in which administrative support services are managed at the AHC level for both the hospital and the medical school. At the University of Massachusetts, for example, the hospital administrator is in name and in fact the vice-chancellor of the medical campus, and services that support the hospital also support the medical school. This does not fully eliminate state influence, but it minimizes difficulty at the medical school or university level. Massachusetts has a separate medical campus at Worcester, away from the main Boston campus; this geographic separateness has simplified some of the problems. At the University of Rochester, the medical campus is in the same city as the main campus. Nevertheless, Strong Memorial Hospital of the University of Rochester is being provided with a similar and growing management capacity at the AHC level.

Perhaps the most interesting solution is the third, in which the university hospital operates in an enterprise mode and support services are purchased from the university. This model is followed at the University of California, San Francisco (UCSF), and Michigan; its success also helps explain why the performance data reported earlier are not more closely correlated with control of support services. William Kerr, Director of Hospitals and Clinics at UCSF, developed the reasons for its success in a recent paper [10]:

> I am convinced that the key to maintaining effective support services is far less a matter of control than it is one of management attention. This is true whether we are focusing on medical, hospital, or general support services. There is clear danger that shared control can generate greater complexity, confusion, and conflict potential. However, there are instances in which the merits of interdependence and integration make these risks well worth taking. And the risks can be minimized by focused management effort. At issue is not who controls, but whether the support service functions in a fashion which is sensitive and responsive to hospital needs.

There are two keys to success in this approach. First is the underlying agreement that the hospital will operate in the enterprise mode; that is, it will be allowed and expected to manage in response to its own mission and the bottom line. Second is the willingness and ability of hospital management to define and then negotiate the agreements which can make these services effective.

This second key to success is not trivial, and may in fact be the more important of the two. We have identified several university hospitals that would have difficulty in following the steps Kerr outlined because of a shortage of talent for the approach he prescribed and interest in it. It is noteworthy that university officers are often less troubled by university hospital initiatives than by university hospital inaction. One university president described a prior administrator as " . . . unequaled in his capacity to analyze any problem into a rationale for inaction." It seems at least possible that one strategy for moving to an enterprise mode is to be enterprising, in precisely the sense that Kerr suggests in the following summary.

STRATEGIES FOR ENSURING RESPONSIVE SUPPORT SERVICES

> First, you must decide how important the support issues are to the effective management of your hospital. Meaningful change will require a real commitment on the part of the hospital's CEO. It is highly unlikely that campus, university, or state officials will consider your concerns a priority if they don't merit your personal involvement.

Having decided that the issue is important, you must determine how things got that way. Are they truly mandated by the state? If developed by the university 20 years ago, are they still appropriate? Accurate determination of the source of difficulty is essential to avoid spinning your wheels. To pinpoint the source you must be conversant with university policies and procedures, state law, and legislative intent. You must also develop a keen understanding of academia.

Next you should prepare a clear, concise plan to approach these issues. If your plan is simply focused on wrestling control from the university or the state, you will most likely find yourself enmeshed in a power struggle. Individual egos, tradition, and job security are at stake. Remember that you cannot solve all of your support service problems simultaneously. Identify those units that have the greatest impact on your hospital operations, and tackle those issues where there is a high likelihood of success. Progress will increase your credibility in both the hospital and university environment.

Having determined those services that merit your immediate and sustained attention, define the characteristics of acceptable performance. Crisp, succinct definition of expectations is essential. As we all know, the best manager, if unaware of the standards by which his performance will be assessed, is likely to fail.

The next step is to share the expectations you have developed with the provider of service. In so doing you should be seeking concurrence that these are reasonable goals. Too often we expect the provider of service to modify operations while we are intractable in our demands. Success will be predicated on having established a true partnership effort, irrespective of who is in control.

Reduce the negotiated agreement to writing, in the form of a contract between the provider and purchaser of services. All salient features regarding performance expectations and costs should be summarized. A management information system that will enable you to track performance must be in place before the plan is implemented. This may be an appropriate point to involve a junior level administrator, working with the support unit to maintain open communications while simultaneously monitoring goal attainment.

At a minimum such service contracts should be reviewed and renewed on an annual basis. They may also require midyear adjustments. We have found annual reassessment involving ultimate approval by the CEO essential to the process. As an aside, we all recognize that contracts documenting the exchange of dollars between units of a common organization have the attendant benefit of substantiating incurred costs for federal and state payers.

Establish user committees for each of the essential service units. At UCSF these committees include representatives from each of the schools, as well as the hospitals and clinics, and serve the purpose of maintaining ongoing dialogue between users and providers of service. Since we support these services through recharge from patient operations, we are extremely sensitive to the cost issue. We have often served as the catalytic agent to initiate expense reduction and improved performance which has benefited the entire campus.

The campus has also developed a program of support unit management effectiveness audits. To avoid the potential adversarial relationship which can evolve when only users evaluate providers, we have called in experts from other university settings to assess the performance of their counterparts. We have found this to be a low-cost, high-yield means of measuring managerial competence, with a side benefit of identifying new programs and methodologies which have succeeded in similar settings.

Capable hospital representatives should be active participants in the selection of all service managers, ranging from clinical department chairmen in the school of medicine to the director of the parking facility. The needs of the hospital are distinctly different from those of the French or microbiology departments of the university. Support service managers must be fully committed to respond appropriately to these unique needs.

CONCLUDING OBSERVATIONS

Several conclusions can be drawn from this investigation of the control of support services in university hospitals:

1. A common belief among university hospital administrators is that gaining control over support services is the answer to the frustration of being held responsible for results they cannot influence. A low degree of hospital control is evident in the administrative support services paralleled in other parts of the university (such as parking, state relations, purchasing, and personnel), but not in patient-related services unique to the hospital (such as pharmacy, social services, patient accounting, and food services).

2. Control over administrative support services occurs at several levels in the hospital's ownership environment. Control at the state level is less common than at the university or AHC level, but its impact can be exacerbated by the university, and in hospitals where state control is substantial it is associated with lower performance. In contrast, control of these services at the hospital or AHC level leads to better hospital performance.

3. Control of these services also leads to better performance when it is not distributed over several different groups. A consequence of multiple control that cannot be quantified is the negative effect it has on the character of hospital administrative work. It tends to force high-level attention on low-level problems, making the jobs less attractive to results-

oriented managers, more attractive to those who rather enjoy bureaucratic infighting. In this way it can shape the roles, and therefore in time, shape the people in these roles.
4. In some settings university-run services *are* responsive to hospital needs. In fact the relatively low correlations between control of support services and performance suggests that control is not the key variable, but simply one of several methods for increasing the responsiveness of these services to hospital needs. Building such responsiveness is not easy when the university will not allow the university hospital to manage its own affairs. Nevertheless, the presence of unresponsive support services at the university level may be an opportunity to help break down that unwillingness, through implementing a rational strategy of making support services responsive to hospital needs. The UCSF experience suggests that, in some university settings, strategic thinking and good management practices can be applied even when support services are in the control of the university.

REFERENCES

1. Westerman, J.H. A requiem for the university hospital? *Health Care Management Review,* 5(Spring 1980):17–24.
2. Dickler, R.M. University hospital finance. Paper presented at Consortium for the Study of University Hospitals Conference, Gainesville, Fla. February 1983.
3. Isaacs, J. *COTH survey of university-owned teaching hospitals' financial and general operating data. 1979, 1980, 1981.* Washington, D.C.: Department of Teaching Hospitals, Association of American Medical Colleges, 1981, 1982, 1983.
4. Mintzberg, H. *The structuring of organizations.* Englewood Cliffs, N.J.: Prentice-Hall, 1979, pp. 288–89.
5. Richards, G. For big-ticket buyers, unity breeds sweeter deal. *Hospitals* 57(December 1, 1983):58–65.
6. Burns, T. *Mechanistic and organismic structures.* In *Organization theory* edited by D.S. Pugh. Baltimore, M.D.: Penguin, 1971.
7. Thompson, J.D. *Organizations in action.* New York: McGraw-Hill, 1967.
8. Pfeffer, J. *Organizational design.* Arlington Heights, Ill.: AHM Publishing Corporation, 1978, pp. 21–24.
9. Chandler, A.D. *Strategy and structure.* Cambridge, Mass.: M.I.T. Press, 1962.
10. Kerr, W.B. Support services. Unpublished paper presented at Consortium for the Study of University Hospitals Conference, Gainesville, Fla., February 24, 1983.

TEN

Medical Staff Organization and Patient Care

All of our previous chapters have discussed the various environments that affect the university hospital. In this chapter we finally focus on the hub of all these variables—patient care. If we think of patient care as a subsystem in our open-systems view of the university hospital, it is the subsystem that acts as the technical core for all of the others. The other subsystems, in fact, provide an artificial external environment that buffers the patient care subsystem from the real environment. So it is important to examine the governance and management of this subsystem.

Although many professional groups provide patient care, our focus here is primarily on the university hospital's medical staff. We are particularly interested in the way in which external pressures—namely, market competition and bureaucratic cost-efficiency controls—have affected the medical staff's provision of patient care.

In this chapter we will first examine how the patient care system is affected by competition and cost controls, both of which vary considerably among hospitals. Secondly, we will examine how the structural forms controlling patient care (including medical service plans and medical staff governance) encourage or inhibit the hospital's response to environmental pressures to compete and control. Finally, we will look beyond formal structures to the more subtle but equally important managerial processes that control patient care.

BACKGROUND

Like other hospitals, university hospitals may be considered "professionalized bureaucracies" in which the medical staff enjoys considerable collective autonomy and monitors its own behavior through the medical staff organization. But unlike the situation in other hospitals, members of the university hospital medical staff are also called "clinical faculty," and are simultaneously members of a similar professional structure within the medical school. This results in dual roles and titles. For example, the chairperson of the internal medicine department within the medical school is typically also the chair or "chief" of the internal medicine division of the university hospital's medical staff. Clearly, there is ample opportunity for these dual roles to give rise to management and governance confusion.

In point of origin, medical schools preceded their associated university hospitals. Universities assisted their medical schools in creating hospitals that would provide patients and facilities for medical faculty, students, and residents to conduct research and receive clinical education. Patient care was always a primary mission, but it was also the means by which the medical school could carry out its research and education missions. In some states, university hospitals were founded to carry out a fourth mission as well—to provide care for indigents.

Knowles characterizes the university hospital's patient care system as having a "balanced biology" [1]. In earlier times when university hospitals were better buffered from the external environment, it was simpler to bring about this balance between the missions. Over the years, however, factors in the institutional environment have caused each of the missions to be emphasized in turn. Until the Flexner report in 1911, patient care was a necessary adjunct of the medical school's educational mission, but somewhat subordinate to it. Beginning with the Flexner report and peaking with the heavy federal funding in the 1950s and 1960s, clinical research was increasingly stressed. These federal funds encouraged the growth of full-time, hospital-based faculty who, in most university hospitals, displaced part-time or volunteer faculty. In the 1960s and early 1970s, federal and state authorities used their funds and influence to expand the size of medical school classes which—together with funding for indigents through Medicaid and the elderly through Medicare—gave rise to a greater emphasis on patient care. As a result, virtually all university hospitals ended the seventies with more clinical faculty and beds than ever before [2,3,4,5,6].

We have already discussed at length the recent changes in governmental policies and funding, and the greater market competition that university hospitals face. These changes have affected the balance among the three missions. The major effect is that clinical faculty spend more time and effort in attracting patients, thus emphasizing patient care. An additional incentive toward emphasis on patient care is the fact that research funding has leveled and dwindled in the past decade, thus eroding this financial base. Finally, prospective reimbursement—at the heart of the DRG system of reimbursement, HMOs, and the newer PPOs (preferred-provider organizations)—is forcing hospitals to stress efficiency and cost control. To summarize, it is clear that hospitals must not only innovate and solve problems in order to compete, they must simultaneously become more efficient in producing routine services.

The two strategic issues for university hospitals—to compete or control—will dictate the structural form of the organization. If the emphasis is on competition, a more organic, self-contained ("product") structure will aid innovation and problem solving. If the emphasis is on efficiency, closing the productive or technical core and instituting a highly bureaucratic, functional and structural form will help control procedures and costs [7,8,9,10]. Clearly, for a patient care system to respond simultaneously to both these environmental pressures requires mutually exclusive structural forms. This is the crux of the organizational problems facing those involved in patient care.

INSTITUTIONAL ENVIRONMENTS

In earlier chapters we provided a detailed explanation of market and political environments. Here, we use that survey data to focus on those aspects of these environments having the greatest relevance to patient care.

As explained in chapter 3, political environments range from those that have proactive state governments (moralistic) to those that have market controls and reactive state governments (traditionalistic). Competitive conditions affecting university hospitals vary from low competition, in which the university hospital enjoys high monopoly power, to intense competition among numerous medical centers in one region. If we consider only the extremes of these two variables, by dichotomizing each of them we have a two-by-two matrix as shown below in figure 10.1.

Figure 10.1 Institutional Environments of University Hospitals

	Market Competition	
Political Environment	Low	High
Moralistic	1.	2.
Traditionalistic	3.	4.

For illustrative purposes, therefore, we could now view university hospitals as facing four possible combinations of market and political environments. However political and market environments are highly related variables, even though they are independent. In reality, politically active states having a moralistic political environment also tend to have highly competitive health markets, and states having a traditional political culture with relatively unbridled competition have less intensely competitive health markets. Consequently, university hospitals do not fall into all of the cells in figure 10.1; instead, most fall into cells 2 and 3. Therefore we can confine our discussion to the environmental conditions in those cells. The data for the discussion is from table 10.1 and from responses in our interviews of physicians and medical administrators.

What does a university hospital medical staff in a cell 2–type environment face? Table 10.1 illustrates the correlation of many variables with this political culture. Typically, this kind of state government makes relatively generous provisions elsewhere for the care of indigents so that the university hospital is not specifically designated as an indigent care hospital. For example in some such states, cities and counties operate separate hospitals for indigents and have relatively generous Medicaid systems for the care of indigents in all hospitals within the state. This reduces outstate referrals of indigents to the university hospital. Intense competition from numerous physician spe-

Table 10.1 Relationship of Political Culture, the Institutional Environment, and the Mission of University Hospitals*

	Correlation Coefficient (r) with Political Culture
Institutional Environment	
State support of welfare (adj. for P.I.)	.61
Urbanization (percent pop. in SMSAs, 1979)	.38
M.D. specialists per 100,000 population	.38
Business climate index	−.40
Percent UH patients from local area	.20
Percent UH patients from outstate areas	−.22
Perceived intensity of local competitive threat	.42
Ownership Environment of the State and University	
Percent university's revenues from research grants	.43
Medical school's rank (based mainly on research rank)	.52
Hospital Mission	
Percent hospital dependence on appropriations (dependence)	−.35
Perceived image of hospital goal of specialty care	.17
Expectation that hospital goal is indigent care	−.24
Perceived image of hospital as indigent care center	−.32
Agreement on hospital goal of tertiary care & research	.25

*A positive (+) sign indicates the variable is correlated positively with a proactive or progressive political climate. A negative (−) sign denotes a conservative, market-oriented political culture.

cialists in regional medical centers throughout the state further reduces these outstate referrals.

The universities in these states mirror these market and political factors in certain ways. These universities are very research oriented and, because of research revenues and endowment income, are less dependent upon state appropriations. Research-oriented universities are associated with research-oriented medical schools. Similarly, universities relatively independent of state appropriations are associated with university hospitals financially independent of the state. These university hospitals do not see themselves as having an indigent care mission. This view is consistent with their not receiving high state appropriations—the latter typically provided as a subsidy for giving care to indigents. Instead these hospitals, mirroring their medical schools, see their mission as providing tertiary care and supporting research by the medical school's clinical faculty.

How do conditions differ in cell 3–type environments? They are just the opposite. Many of these hospitals were founded with an indigent care mission and receive high state appropriations. Being less research oriented, their universities rely much more heavily on state appropriations. Similarly their medical schools are less research oriented. Fortunately, market conditions for these hospitals tend to be more benign because the state has fewer regional medical centers and physician specialists. Consequently, these university hospitals receive more outstate referrals.

Members of the medical staff in one cell 3–type environment presented the following picture of what they face when they try to compete. Since their state has relatively few regional medical centers, this university hospital should have been able to attract referrals. However, it was founded as an indigent care center for the state, and continues to have that image; furthermore, it is heavily subsidized for providing indigent care. As a result, its indigent-care image inhibits the attraction of private paying patients and referrals on a medical rather than financial basis. The medical staff wants to turn this situation around by competing vigorously, but to do so would incur the wrath of private physicians.

Why has this happened? The staff explained the interesting but politically frustrating situation. According to our respondents, private hospitals, particularly corporate chains, have "broken the planning laws" by building, leasing, and buying hospitals throughout the state. This procompetition climate encourages competition in private health care but, paradoxically, has acted against the university hospital. All respondents agreed that if university hospital physicians were to move aggressively to market their services and otherwise compete, it would be viewed as unfair competition by government against private enterprise!

Over and over throughout the interviews around the country, physicians have complained that their ties with government prevent their competing. Unfortunately, the transition in the 1960s to full-time, hospital-based staffs in university hospitals, financed primarily by generous research funding and capitation funds from the federal government, has in effect made university hospital staffs competitors with private physicians—some of whom are still chafing about losing their status as volunteer faculty.

These pressures are, of course, much greater for state university-owned hospitals. If local physicians object to competition from a private university-owned hospital, they can retaliate by reducing their referrals, but if this occurs with a state university-owned hospital, physicians can also bring pressure to bear on politicians and state officials. Respondents indicated that the threat is greatest in the area of primary and family practice care. (Obviously, a university hospital medical staff competes with fewer superspecialist physicians in tertiary-level care than with physicians in the lower levels of care.)

Although most university hospital physicians face opposition from private physicians to their competition, the situation is not quite as difficult in hospitals in cell 2–type environments. There are three major differences. First, there are many more major-medical-center hospitals in these environments with which university hospitals are already competing; therefore, whatever a university hospital and its medical staff do competitively is neither as noticeable nor as influential as it would be in the less competitive cell 3–type environment. Second, the more research-oriented hospital in the cell 2–type environment is likely to be moving into some new area on the frontiers of medical science, not merely duplicating services provided by its competitors. Third, a hospital in a cell 2–type environment is less dependent upon state appropriations and is consequently less subject to financial (political) pressures from state and university officials. Finally, because it is not viewed as a quasi-state agency, it has greater freedom to compete.

Structure: Medical Service Plans (MSPs)

In our investigation of how university hospitals respond to the environmental pressures to compete for and control patient-care services, we consider the university hospital's organizational responses in two ways. First, we will examine how the medical staff has changed its structure at the operational level. Next we will discuss changes at the policy or strategic level with the advent of MSPs, where coordination and collaboration occur between top officials of the medical staff, hospital administration, the medical school, other schools within the health sciences center, and the university.

Medical care has traditionally been provided by fee-for-service, solo practitioners, and has always had an entrepreneurial character. In recent decades, these physicians have increasingly joined group-practice arrangements because of the economies of scale involved in assembling the expensive equipment and personnel required for private practice, together with a variety of other group-practice benefits (such as rotating on call).

Historically, clinical faculty in university hospitals enjoyed no such flexibility. After World War II they became full-time, salaried employees of university hospitals, and their income as a result was subject to real pressures. We have already explained in this chapter how the patient load has increased in the last few decades; despite this increase, there were no organizational incentives required to encourage clinical faculty to increase their emphasis on patient care. If, for example, a salaried physician were to give more care, it had no effect on his personal income. To remedy this, the more prominent faculty were often permitted to maintain some beds for their "private" patients—the income from the latter being incremental income beyond their salary. The usual effect of this device was to sow seeds of discord among the faculty not enjoying this privilege.

In some university hospitals, faculty had admitting privileges in one or more community hospitals to which they would admit their nonteaching patients. In this arrangement, the university hospital tended to receive a disproportionately large share of the indigents, while the community hospitals received more than their share of paying patients and those with the interesting medical diagnoses. University hospitals, wanting to attract the better clinicians, and the medical schools, wanting to attract the best clinical faculty, found it increasingly difficult to compete against the salaries available in private practice. To make it even worse—in a few situations—if the clinical faculty were able to generate surplus, unencumbered funds, the state would confiscate them. In such cases the state argued that current surpluses were available to repay the state for having provided subsidies to faculty and the university hospital in the past. Hence, if clinical faculty were successful, they faced the loss of the fruits of their labors.

Consequently, in the early 1970s clinical faculties began forming various group-practice arrangements that have become known by the generic title of medical practice or service plans (MSPs). Definitive data concerning the total volume of their annual fee billings are not available, but they will undoubtedly be about one billion dollars in 1984 [11,12,13]. An MSP is a mechanism for collecting fees and distributing them in prearranged proportions among physicians, clinical department heads, the medical school dean, and sometimes other parties or special funds. There are four salient structural features of MSPs, as explained below: faculty composition and academic purpose, administrative structure, arrangements for controlling revenues and disbursements, and financial incentives [14,15].

1. *Faculty.* MSPs are an arrangement for a medical school's clinical faculty whose missions include research and education. Therefore, in university-owned institutions, their ultimate ac-

countability is to the university; they are not an autonomous, separate entity.

2. *Administrative structure.* Rather than merely an added function of the medical school structure, an MSP is a separately governed administrative structure which often mirrors the medical staff structure. If the hospital is a principal affiliate of the university rather than owned by it, the MSP structure is needed to form independent practitioners into a group practice. However in university-owned hospitals the clinical faculty already have the medical school structure forming them into a group practice. It is unusual, therefore, for physicians in the latter setting to set up an MSP as a separate legal entity independent of medical school control.

3. *Controlling revenues and disbursements.* An MSP involves a plan for salaries, fees, collections, and disbursements by which group criteria and decisions replace the individual discretion of physicians. Individual earnings are pooled by section, department, or school.

4. *Incentives.* An MSP redistributes professional fee earnings in order to achieve faculty goals. Hence the chest surgeon may earn little more than the pediatrician because the chest surgeon's earnings may be used to subsidize the pediatrician. Similarly, senior physicians' earnings are used to subsidize basic science faculty and junior members of the clinical faculty. This is done by negotiating the total and component parts of each member's salary and the distribution of surpluses and subsidies remaining in the pool.

To keep faculty from ignoring patient care, the plan may allow them to retain a significant portion of the fee income they generate. Conversely, to keep faculty from overly stressing patient care, a salary cap may be set at the beginning of the year; professional fees earned beyond that are placed in the MSP pool. To encourage research, a physician might be given a guarantee of $90,000 ($30,000 from the state for teaching, and $30,000 cap on professional fee income) with the additional $30,000 required to come from research generated by the physician.

Surpluses are not only routinely generated under these arrangements, they are built into the calculations. Although the physicians generating these surpluses generally retain a fraction of earnings over their target cap, the greater part is normally retained in the section, department, or medical school pool. Typically, the dean receives for the school some fixed percentage—around 10 percent. This is widely known as the "Dean's tax."

The distribution of these surpluses and subsidies provides considerable leverage or power overlaying the formal control structure. A department chairman presiding over an unencumbered pool of millions of dollars within a financially impoverished setting can wield considerable influence.

Control is important. MSPs capture patient-care income; successful MSPs capture a great deal of it. MSPs supplement the university's reward system as it operates in the medical school; successful MSPs support the ideal balance of research, teaching, and service that the medical school wishes to achieve. These two definitions of success—income and balanced mission—are not easily meshed, and contests for control can easily arise between the faculty that generates the revenues and the administration obligated to direct the use of those revenues.

For example, one source of conflict is the amount that an "independent" MSP must pay for the use of hospital space. As the market becomes more competitive, the clinical faculty are increasing their demands for status as a separate legal entity and the freedom to lease or own clinic facilities exempt from hospital or university overhead charges. A potential solution is the return of the two-clinic system. In this system, private practice is conducted in MSP-controlled clinics leased from the hospital at market rates, and poorer patients failing the "green (means) test" are treated in the hospital's clinics where resident education occurs.

The solution that would best meet the needs of the university and be least threatening to the competition and the state would be to balance the missions of care, research, and education. In practical terms, this means clinical faculty would derive about one-third of their total income from each of these three sources. By so doing, they would spend less time in competing against community physicians for health-care dollars, and more time in research and education. To meet the research objective, and to some extent the teaching objective, the medical faculty needs a specific type of patient (usually advanced tertiary-care patients). Thus the emphasis on research rather than competition has systematic effects on all three missions. To attain a balance between the three missions, the university itself would have to provide a supportive research environment—for example, critical support and administrative services to obtain grants, to allocate research space, provide seed money for research projects, and allocate research assistants.

In sum, a benign and supportive university environment is paramount to achieving a balance between the three missions, because support for education will not come from patient-care dollars. It is clear that such an environment is becoming more scarce. Competitive patient care is a reality forcing the university hospital and its clinical faculty to choose among much less pleasant alternatives.

Structure: Medical Staff Governance

Having looked at some of the structural responses at the operating level, we turn now to examine the nature of governance-level structure for the patient care subsystem. This structure has undergone an evolutionary change since university hospitals were founded as clinical laboratories of medical schools. Typically, these early university hospitals were operated by numerous medical school officials according to the particular structure of the medical school. Medical school department heads, in their capacity as chiefs of the corresponding hospital services, ran these hospital units as largely autonomous units. Nonprofessional support services, clerical, and administrative affairs were often shoved aside under a less powerful business manager. This model, known as the "strong dean" model, typically progressed until one associate dean was given authority over all hospital affairs [16,17]. This model survives today primarily in private university-owned university hospitals.

As university hospitals became larger, more complex, more financially independent, and more oriented toward third-party payers, the administrative load overwhelmed medical school administration. Consequently, the hospital was taken out of the medical school and placed under the control of a hospital director reporting to a university official. In this model, known as the "bicameral" model, the university hospital director is in theory a peer of the medical school dean. The medical school dean reports with other deans through the education-research hierarchy, which in a university is of course the line hierarchy. The university hospital is a support function in the university setting, and its director may report to more than one vice-president as well as a provost or president. This imbalance in formal authority and prestige and absence of a common superior to coordinate their affairs can cause and has caused various kinds of frictions and administrative difficulties.

Given the high interdependence between medical school and hospitals, however, university officials and committees are not the primary means of coordination. Routine execution of JCAH (Joint Commission on the Accreditation of Hospitals) standards and guidelines are typically handled by standing committees of the medical staff. In contrast, nonroutine matters—those involving critical matters and politically charged issues such as allocating beds, expanding or contracting services, and large capital equipment purchases—are generally handled by the executive committee of the medical staff, by numerous conferences among the dean, the director, and their associates, and by advice from the joint conference committee of the board or its equivalent.

A major problem with the bicameral model is the question, "Who has overall responsibility for the quality of medical care?" Under the strong-dean model, the dean is clearly both responsible for care and in control of the care process. But under the bicameral model, with medical school faculty and hospital medical staff separated, the dean no longer has direct control of the practice of medicine within the university hospital. Legally, the dean as dean cannot be responsible for patient care, because this responsibility rests with the university hospital governing authorities and their delegates—including the medical staff and university hospital director.

Some university hospitals have solved this by giving the dean the responsibility. However, the manner in which the dean controls the medical staff in order to fulfill the responsibilities is much more problematic than a simple legal mandate would imply. The dean always has indirect control through the power to appoint medical school faculty and chairpersons, which generally determines as well the corresponding administrative positions within the hospital. The dean can also directly control the medical staff by being on key hospital committees, possibly being on the university hospital board, and by simply supervising the chief of staff (COS), also known as the medical director.

This COS role is generally appointed rather than elected, is theoretically a part-time position but is really full time, and has as its principal function to be the liaison between the medical staff, medical school, and university hospital administration [18,19,20,21]. In reality, we have found this role to be ambiguous. No two COS roles are the same; all of the chiefs of staff define their role as they execute it, and seem to be somewhat uncertain of their formal powers. Like factory foremen, they are "in the middle," that is, not fully managers and no longer fully mere workers [22]. The COS's role varies depending on method of appointment, reporting lines, memberships, and formal powers. Typically the COS is jointly appointed by the dean and the director. The COS may carry a dual title such as Associate Dean of the Medical School for Clinical Affairs and be paid by both the university hospital and the medical school. As COS he reports to the university hospital director; as associate dean he reports to the dean.

In practice, however, these formal structural features do not accurately describe the real role of the COS. This role is evolving, being formed in the breach created by separating administration of the hospital from the medical school. The particular nature of the role has been determined by a multitude of variables within each situation—including personalities—which are not captured by the simple characteristics of formal structure, such as who appoints and who pays. We have seen associate deans as chiefs of staff who define their role as liaison for the university hospital director to the dean, and we have seen medical directors, appointed and wholly paid by the university hospital director, who see their role as either the medical staff's advocate or "the Dean's man" in the hospital.

These difficulties in coordinating the university hospital and medical school have caused the parties involved to seek coordination from the "bureaucratic higher-ups"—in this case, university vice-presidents or presidents. These administrations, already swamped with responsibility, have typically appointed a single, new vice-president over the university hospital, the medical school, and typically all other health-related schools and colleges [23]. This role is known by various titles, the most frequent being the vice-president for health affairs (VPHA), and the model is known as the "corporate" model.

The power of the VPHA depends on how much power other vice-presidents of the university give up. For example, the vice-president for financial affairs must give up some control over personnel, purchasing, stores, labor relations, and general accounting within the university hospital and the health-related schools on campus. The vice-president for academic affairs (or provost on some campuses) must likewise give up some control over appointments, promotions, and salaries of faculty in the medical school.

For two reasons we have not emphasized in this discussion the role of the hospital board. Our primary reason is that it has been discussed separately in chapter 3. Just as important, however, is the fact that some type of hospital board must exist within each of the three models just discussed. Guidelines of JCAH mandate the existence of a hospital board that controls the quality of medical care, and all university hospitals have them regardless of their model of governance. Where hospital boards are separate from both medical school and university governance, they have typically begun as dependent bodies dealing primarily with controlling the quality of care and over time expanded their purview into medico-administrative matters. For example, the regents of the university may begin as the official university hospital board, but for practical purposes university hospital governance is handled by a committee of the regents that includes hospital and medical school representatives as well as—in some cases—representatives of the community. As the administrative burden as well as their competence has increased, they have been given a role in university hospital governance. The theoretical limit of this evolutionary process is for the university to set this university hospital board outside the university structure, and this has rarely been done.

As mentioned in the introduction to this chapter, the twin strategic issues of competition and cost control have strained the governance structures we have just described, because these issues call for opposing structures for the patient-care subsystem. Competition calls for a more organic structure in order to encourage problem solving and innovation; conversely, efficiency calls for a more mechanistic structure. Since both situations occur simultaneously, the recommended course of action is unclear. In theory an organization can face such incompatible demands sequentially, or it can have separate parts of the organization each deal with only one of the environmental demands. In this case, the patient-care subsystem must deal with both, and deal with them simultaneously.

If university hospitals had either a functional or a product-type structure, the structural response to these environmental demands would be simpler. If they were totally functional in structure, they could become more competitive by creating better horizontal linkages, (for example through task forces and liaison roles). Most hospitals are in fact functionally structured; the University of Michigan Hospital system is an example. The only exceptions within this structure are specialty clinics, such as children's or psychiatric clinics. These remain somewhat outside of the main structure.

On the other hand, if university hospitals were totally structured into self-contained or product-type groups, they could be more efficient and control cost by horizontal linkages along functional lines [24]. For example, Johns Hopkins Hospital comes as close to having a product-type structure as any teaching hospital [25]. Here many of the typical supporting functions in a patient-care unit are administratively a part of the unit. However, certain functions like pathology and radiology units are centralized. If the new DRG system of reimbursement places pressures on JHH to monitor the ordering of certain test procedures and reduce the expense of providing these procedures, to do so would require coordination along functional lines (pathology, radiology) which, given the product-type structure of Johns Hopkins Hospital, would mean coordination across the various self-contained patient care services.

In fact, all university hospitals are hybrid, or matrix structures, within university structures that are similarly hybrid. In any hospital, the patient care unit is a matrix in that physicians, by means of their medical orders on the patient's chart, exert strong control over and coordination of the various separate functional departments represented on the patient unit [26]. For example, nursing, housekeeping, and dietary all have personnel in every patient's room every day. Employees of each of these three functional departments are subject to the authority of their respective functional bosses and to the orders of the physician. Most university hospitals have a mixture of these functional and product-type structures. For example, if a children's or woman's hospital has a separate administrator and includes enough functions to make it virtually self-contained, this is a product-type division. However, every university hospital has some centralized functions at the corporate level such as labor relations, legal, and public relations. Hence, employees within a children's hospital are subject to redundant, crisscrossing lines of authority—making the overall structure a hybrid or matrix.

The combination of these factors makes each university hospital structure unique and precludes simple conclusions about how its formal structure has been altered to respond to strategic contingencies within the environment. What we did observe is that power is diffuse—which is the essence and intent of hybrid and matrix structures. Our measures of power over various decisions closely related to patient care are reported by role in table 10.2. The higher the score, the more influence the official sanctioned by that position has in a decision.

Clearly, there is no simple bureaucratic hierarchy in operation here, as evidenced by the fact that the chief (equivalent to department chairman within the medical school) is more influential than the VPHA or the dean in most categories. There is faint evidence of the well-known dual hierarchy operating here, in that chiefs and the dean have greater power in the highly professional area of determining appointments and privileges of physicians, and the two bureaucratic officials in the administrative hierarchy (the VPHA and the hospital administrator) have greater authority in functions of a less professional nature like allocating space and paying house staff.

With the data in table 10.2 we attempted to determine if any one role clearly dominated within any of the university hospitals. We decided to identify those hospitals in which the aggregate power of one of the officials is clearly dominant across all six decisions. We found that there are few cases in which either the dean or the VPHA is dominant; therefore, we combined these two offices to form a single category, which we labeled "centralized." Table 10.3 shows the types of patient-care control structures that result. If no decision maker dominated, we labeled it a "federation" structure in which power is diffuse. If chiefs were dominant, we considered this to be relatively "decentralized."

What is at once obvious in table 10.3 is that a large proportion of

Table 10.2 Influence over Patient Care–Related Decisions

	Governance Officials			Management
	VPHA	Dean	Chief	Hospital Administrator
Expanding, contracting services	2.5	1.8	3.0	2.7
Allocating space	1.8	1.3	1.7	2.9
Setting future direction, emphasis on research	2.1	2.4	2.7	1.6
Determine appointments, privileges	1.4	1.8	2.8	1.3
How house staff, residents paid	1.7	1.6	1.5	2.5
Allocating beds by service	1.5	1.3	2.3	2.7
Average	1.83	1.7	2.33	2.28

Note: 0 = minor, no influence; 3 = major, decisive influence.

Table 10.3 Patient Care Control Structures

	N	%
VPHA/dean (centralized)	10	18
Chiefs (decentralized)	24	44
Federation (diffuse)	21	38
	55	100

university hospitals have no clear locus of control in the area of decisions crucial to patient care. Almost two-fifths have "diffuse" structures, with no dominant structural form.

Our attempts to find linkages between the political and market environments and types of patient-care control structures were predictably disappointing. Few patterns appear. There is a slight tendency for moralistic political cultures with high market competition to be associated with a more decentralized control structure by the chiefs, and for traditional political environments with low market competition to be associated with federation control, but the correlations are not strong. Similarly, there are only weak linkages between types of patient-care control structure and measures of performance in the areas of patient care, research, and education.

University hospitals are characterized by complex rather than simple structure, and different formal structures (centralized, diffuse, decentralized) apparently handle similar environmental demands equally well. Clues to better performance will derive more from the informal structure for decision making than from formal structure. This decision-making process is the subject of the next section.

MANAGEMENT PROCESS: CLARITY IN DECISION MAKING

The inconclusiveness of our analysis of survey data in locating patterns between environment and structure was offset by four conclusions flowing from the interviews. First, when nonroutine decisions are made, the formal structure is less crucial than the informal decision-making pathways within it. Formal structures guide routine responses to routine contingencies, whereas responses to current competitive and regulatory pressures are nonroutine demands better handled in an ad hoc manner.

Second, the type of environmental contingency—competition for patients or pressure on costs—does not dictate centralization or level at which decisions are made, or success in dealing with the problem. Certain aspects of given decisions must be handled at lower levels and other aspects of the same decisions at higher levels, but few problems are addressed exclusively at one or the other extremes.

Third, as many experts in organization behavior have said, power is not a fixed commodity or zero-sum phenomenon in university hospitals [27]. In our field studies of university hospitals, those that seemed to us to be better have strong leaders and institutions at *all* levels. Typically a strong patient care system is associated with strong department chairpersons and strong leadership within the hospital, medical school, and university. We have seen exceptions to strong leadership at higher levels, but never exceptions to strong department leaders (clinical chiefs). The more typical situation, however, is strong leaders at several levels. We interviewed individuals enjoying a national reputation for being "autocratic" leaders, and found that in fact they use participative management among a set of strong leaders. As in any organization, strong leaders in patient-care systems reflect strong leadership within the university and the medical school, and themselves attract equally strong leaders as clinical chiefs.

Fourth, and most important, clarity in decision making is more crucial than purity of organization structure. Clarity does not imply any particular organizational form, for many forms seem to work. Instead, clarity is a combination of three factors.

1. The number of key decision makers, which ranges from a dominant individual, to a ruling oligarchy, to a collegial body or legislature.
2. The method of decision making, which ranges along one dimension from explicit or formal means to ad hoc, implicit, political coalition building.
3. Knowledge of the system, which ranges from a good understanding of the true nature of who makes decisions and how they are made, to lack of knowledge, to misinformation.

The second and third variables, method (or formality) and knowledge, are conceptually distinct, but in typical practice they are closely related: formal systems are often well-understood systems. Therefore these two variables are treated here as one, and their combination with the first variable produces the two-by-two matrix shown in figure 10.2.

In our field studies we observed all four types of decision or control structures shown in figure 10.2. Executive and collegial types of structures both seem to work reasonably well, even though they are quite different approaches. In the executive approach, there are a few key decision makers rather than just one. This does not mean that the same decision makers make all decisions: those who are key to a particular decision vary by issue, and a key attribute of good leadership here is to be judicious in routing decisions to the right persons. In a collegial approach, decisions are routed to the appropriate bodies—the groups involved varying by issue. The common factor among these two is their predictability and workability: decisions are made expeditiously because most persons know how and where they will be made.

The other two modes of decision making, by dominant individuals and shifting coalitions, do not seem to work as well. They are less common in the university hospitals we thought were well managed and successful. The dominant personality approach differs from the executive approach in that the former personalities are dominant in all decisions, whereas in the latter, influence shifts to those having knowledge relevant to a given decision. Likewise, the political model differs from the collegial model in that the former has no predictable membership or decision pathway, and influence seems to flow to those skilled in manipulation rather than to those with knowledge relevant to a particular decision.

Figure 10.2 Clarity of Control Structure

| | Number of Decision Makers | |
How Decisions Made	Few	Many
Well understood, formal	Executive or bureaucratic	Collegial or legislative
Not well understood, informal, ad hoc	Dominant personalities	Political, diffuse

CONCLUSION

University hospitals are being influenced by the twin issues of competition and efficiency. Competition demands a more organic, decentralized structure given to innovative ways of attracting and retaining patients. Certainly clinical chiefs and faculty must be involved in marketing university hospital services—in fact, they ought to be good at it. The move in the past decade toward MSPs has provided the incentives and organizational framework for clinicians to be leaders in the marketing of their patient care services.

The environment is also forcing administrators to be more efficient in providing care services. More efficient production requires a more mechanistic, centralized structure—exactly the opposite of what innovative marketing requires. The patient-care system is essentially a self-contained or product-type structure, created for ease in dealing with the market environment; in contrast, the administrative structure overlaying patient care is typically a functional structure. This combination of product and functional structures produces a hybrid or matrix-type structure in university hospitals, which makes it possible for them to respond to simultaneous and incompatible demands from the environment such as market pressures and cost pressures.

The hybrid structure controlling the patient-care system encourages the diffusion of power among many roles and decision groups, and cannot be characterized by the simple notion of centralization. Looking solely at centralization, there are few clear patterns between environmental demands and the university hospital's structure for controlling patient care or its performance outcomes. Those patterns important to effective patient care are the managerial processes or informal decision processes within the formal structure.

The key that emerged from the interviews is the necessity of having strong leaders and institutions at all levels. First, it is especially important to have strong clinical chiefs (department chairpersons). Secondly, clarity in decision making is important. Regardless of whether few or many are involved in decisions and whether they are at lower or higher levels in the hierarchy, it is important that they have appropriate knowledge and interest in order to make the decisions, and that the procedure for routing the decision to them is reasonable and predictable. This is understandable in light of the issues and structures we have analyzed. Simultaneous environmental demands requiring mutually exclusive structures are confronting a decentralized, organic patient care system embedded within a mechanistic, centralized administrative structure. This can be a prescription either for a patient-care control structure that is in a muddle or, if clarity is present, one that can respond effectively.

REFERENCES

1. Knowles, J.H. The balanced biology of the teaching hospital. *New England Journal of Medicine* 269(1963):401–55.
2. Isaacs, J. *COTH survey of university-owned teaching hospitals' financial and general operating data. 1979, 1980, 1981.* Washington, D.C.: Department of Teaching Hospitals, Association of American Medical Colleges, 1981, 1982, 1983.
3. Thomas, J. Datagram: Income analysis of university-owned teaching hospitals. *Journal of Medical Education* 52(1977):528–31.
4. Schramm, C.J. The teaching hospital and the future role of state government. *New England Journal of Medicine* 308(1983):41–45.
5. Fredrickson, D.S. Biomedical research in the 1980s. *New England Journal of Medicine* 304(1981):509–17.
6. Rogers, D.E., and R.J. Blendon. The academic medical center: A stressed american institution. *New England Journal of Medicine* 298(1978): 940–50.
7. Charns, M.P. Breaking the tradition barrier: Managing integration in health care facilities. *Health Care Management Review* 1(Winter, 1976):55–67.
8. Sayles, L.R. Matrix management: The structure with a future. *Organizational Dynamics* 5(Autumn 1976):2–17.
9. Hunt, R.G. Technology and organization. *Academy of Management Journal* 13(1970):235–52.
10. Burns, T., and G.M. Stalker. *The management of innovation.* London: Tavistock, 1961.
11. Hilles, W.C., and S.K. Fagan. *Medical practice plans at U.S. medical schools: A review of current characteristics and trends. Vol. I (Interim Final*

Report). Washington, D.C.: Association of American Medical Colleges, 1977.
12. Relman, A.S. Faculty-practice plans. *New England Journal of Medicine.* 304(1981):292–93.
13. Siegel, B. Medical service plans in academic medical centers. *Journal of Medical Education* 53(1978):791–98.
14. Kasonic, J. Oral presentation, August 8, 1979.
15. Stein, R.M. Oral presentation, 1980.
16. Wilson, M.P., R.M. Knapp, and A.B. Jones. The growing managerial imperative of the academic medical center. In *Health management for tomorrow,* edited by S. Levy and T. McCarthy. Philadelphia: J.B. Lippincott Co., 1980, pp. 81–108.
17. Petersdorf, R.G., and M.P. Wilson. The four horsemen of the apocalypse. *Journal of the American Medical Association* 247(1982):1153–61.
18. Williams, K.J. The role of the medical director. *Hospital Progress* 59(June 1978):50–57.
19. Shortell, S., and C. Evashwick. The structural configuration of U.S. hospital medical staffs. *Medical Care* 19(1981):419–30.
20. Lloyd, J.S. Medical directors grow in numbers, responsibilities. *The Hospital Medical Staff* 12(February 1983):12–19.
21. Rogatz, P. The evolving role of the medical director. *The Hospital Medical Staff* 10(October 1981):14–19.
22. Dubin, R., et al. *Leadership and productivity.* San Francisco: Chandler Publishing Co., 1965, pp. 114–32.
23. Hogness, J.R., and G.C. Akin. Administration of education programs in academic health centers. *New England Journal of Medicine* 296(1977): 656–88.
24. Sayles, L.R., and R.L. Daft. In *Organization theory and design,* by R.L. Daft. St. Paul, Minn.: West Publishing Co., 1983, chap. 6.
25. Solomon, S. How one hospital broke its inflation fever. *Fortune* 99 (April–June, 1979):148–54.
26. Neuhauser, D. The hospital as a matrix organization. *Hospital Administration* 17 (Fall 1972):8–25.
27. Tannenbaum, A.S. *Control and organization.* New York: McGraw-Hill, 1968.

ELEVEN

Governance and Management of University Hospitals

The three sets of management issues of finance, support services, and patient care produce the governance problem for university hospitals. This chapter will move away from the focus on specific issues of the three preceding chapters to the problem of managing and governing the hospital as a whole.

SUMMARY OBSERVATIONS

It is helpful to begin with five summary observations:

1. State government influence on some university hospitals is pronounced, and from the hospital's and university's perspective has only one thing to commend it—it helps somewhat to keep state appropriations and other support high [1]. However, its effect on efficiency of operations and on quality of governance and management of university hospitals is negative. In states with an activist orientation, the problem of state control is smaller or less common, and the possibility of reducing it is much better.

2. University influence on most hospitals is still strong, and has several things to commend it [2].
   a. It helps protect the financial position of the parent university.
   b. It helps somewhat in keeping state appropriations high.
   c. It helps in keeping a strong teaching, or teaching-research emphasis in hospital decision making.

   However its effect on efficiency of operations, and on quality of management of university hospitals, is negative.

3. A university tends to want to increase control over the hospital in order to manage the growing complexity of the health education enterprise, and because the state is less willing to fund full university and hospital appropriations requirements [3]. In contrast, a hospital wants to lessen university control because of growing competition for patients and growing complexity of regulations [4]. These two incompatible pressures account for a significant part of the hospital governance problem.

4. A possible solution to these twin problems is to give the hospital autonomy by channeling all significant influence (from the state government, the university administration, the medical school, the community) through a strong governing board, and to give the university control through its control of membership on that board. One or both parts of this logic helps explain the rapid rise of university hospital governing boards in the past 15 years.

5. Such a crystallization of power is likely to strengthen the role of hospital administration and to weaken the influence of other groups. This helps explain why many of these hospital boards have not gained, or been given, power [5].

Setting for the Governance Problem

There are several groups that have an important stake in the hospital: the medical school, university, community, state government, and hospital administration [6]. These are defined broadly below, omitting important qualifications.

University

The university has a strong interest in hospital performance, both to protect the university's integrity and to preserve that source of university prestige. In fact, it has the strongest of all claims, asserted through legal ownership.

Medical School

The medical school also has a strong interest in hospital performance, to support the function of teaching and research. It has an historic claim, for university hospitals were for the most part started for this purpose. It has a strong power base, for the hospital's primary distinctiveness rests on its staffing by the clinical faculty and its rich resource of residents.

It is often useful to distinguish between two of the components that make up this group, the medical school's administration and the clinical chiefs. The clinical chiefs are central to the success of the teaching-research-patient care enterprise, and as a result have substantial power. The growing importance of patient care as a source of revenue creates stresses within the medical school, and may link the interests of the chiefs more closely to the hospital as the producer of patient care, than to the university and medical school as an educational institution.

State Government

The state government has no clear interest in hospital performance distinct from the two above, with the exception of a minor though troublesome interest in bureaucratic control of procedures for the purpose of equity, economy, or detection of wrongdoing. In some settings, the state may have a strong interest in using the hospital to care for indigents.

Community

The community has a weak interest in hospital performance. Though it pays for and receives the care rendered, health care needs may often be met elsewhere. It also exerts the weakest claim because "community" here describes an aggregation and not an organized interest group. Its potential power is great, but it is exercised through an impersonal market and political processes which cannot easily be harnessed in support of a claimant. University hospitals are considered a statewide resource, but state residents provide them no organized constituency. Although located within a local community that could provide support, local patients do not see university hospitals as existing for them. Moreover, some local hospitals see them as a competitive threat.

Hospital Administration

Hospital administration does not bring independent interests to controlling the hospital. However, it does have a strong interest in making it a fit instrument for achieving some viable set of the interests described above. Its power base lies in its capacity to organize and facilitate, turning disparate parts into a productive system and identifying sources of necessary resources.

"Governance" is the process of controlling the hospital, to ensure that it does achieve some viable set of the interests described above. One may say that the state, university, medical school, and community have an interest in the outcomes of governance, but, assuming the outcomes are generally acceptable, less interest in the governance process itself. Hospital administration has a strong interest in the process of governance but less in whose interests are served—so long as interests are consistent with each other, and with the hospital's continued viability.

Framing the Questions: The Influence of Key Groups and Hospital Performance

Our purpose in this chapter is to present data on the distribution of influence among the key groups in the university hospital's ownership environment, and to show the relation that this power distribution has to hospital performance. First, we present data that link key management variables with the level of state appropriations, and review the findings reported in chapter 7—that increased competitive pressure does not appear to be related to a stronger external orientation by hospital management—in the context of the possible influence of the university hospital's ownership environment. The chapter concludes with a discussion of four organizational structures that accommodate and reflect different influence distributions among key groups in the ownership environment of the university hospital, and reasons why some may prove more desirable than others in the future.

Data on the distribution of influence among key groups is drawn from the CSUH survey described in chapter 3. The measures of performance are those viability and efficiency indexes described in chapter 4, and the measure for state appropriation is defined in table 7.1 of chapter 7. Three of the four variables used in this chapter to describe university hospital management and governance have not been used before in this book. All are described below.

— *AHC/hospital board.* Of the eight identifiable types of hospital governance bodies reported in the CSUH survey, two types—the hospital board and the academic health center board—operated close to or at the hospital level, were formal bodies, and together made up 37 percent of all hospitals reporting. For this variable, hospitals with an AHC or hospital board were assigned a "1," those with some other form of governance were assigned a "0."

— *Board external orientation.* Survey respondents indicated one of four areas in which their board functioned most effectively. In scaling these, we identified "externally oriented" boards as those that left management to hospital executives and focused board efforts on obtaining resources from the environment, negotiating with it, and protecting the hospital from it. We identified "internally oriented" boards as those that focused on setting the hospital's direction through long-range planning and in assisting management. The scale had four values, ranging from a strong internal to a strong external orientation (see chapter 3, table 3.8).

— *HA/board power.* This variable combines influence data for the hospital board and the hospital administration columns of the decision-making power question, using data from all 14 decision areas (see chapter 3, table 3.10).

— *External management orientation.* The data for this variable come from a survey question that asked respondents to report on a four-point scale the amount of high-level administration attention required for each of a dozen external groups, including third-party payers, regulatory and review agencies, and other health care organizations. We used this data to index the external orientation of the hospital's management.

Findings

An initial analysis of the data on influence addressed its distribution among key groups by different types of decisions. The results are shown in tables 11.1, 11.2 and 11.3. The data show an expected pattern. For example, the trustees and hospital-board group have their greatest influence in governance and finance, and their least influence in management and patient care. University officials have their least influence in patient care, where the dean and chiefs have the greatest. Hospital administration has its greatest influence in management and support services, its least in governance and patient care.

It is important to emphasize the influence of medical school administration and the clinical chiefs on patient-care management decisions. These are policy-administrative, not clinical decisions (which of course are the domain of individual physicians). Our data indicate that in most university hospitals, the management of the core mission of

Table 11.1 Average Influence for Governance Groups in Selected Decision Categories (in Percents)

Decision Category	Group			
	Trustees and Hospital Board	University Officials and VPHA	Medical School Administration and Clinical Chiefs	Hospital Administration
All decisions	16	29	30	26
Governance	22	32	28	18
Management	11	26	32	34
Patient care	11	19	48	22
Finance	24	33	19	24
Support	13	31	16	40

Table 11.2 Influence of Governance Bodies and Administration on Governance Decisions

Governance Decisions	Influence (%)		Influence (Rank in 14 Decisions)	
	Trustees and Hospital Board	Hospital Administration	Trustees and Hospital Board	Hospital Administration
Reorganization at the governance level to give substantial autonomy to the university hospital	30	12	1	12
Decisions on amount and sources of capital financing (e.g., borrowing)	30	18	2	9
Fund raising (philanthropic)	22	16	3	10
Choose and/or appoint a new hospital administrator	20	8	4	14
Decisions on capital budget allocations	20	26	5	6
Future directions, and emphasis on clinical research*	6	16	12	11

*Patient care decision.

Table 11.3 Influence of Governance Bodies and Administration on Operating Decisions

Operating Decisions	Influence (%)		Influence (Rank in 14 Decisions)	
	Trustees and Hospital Board	Hospital Administration	Trustees and Hospital Board	Hospital Administration
Reorganization of hospital management (e.g., decentralization) to place accountability with second-level managers.	8	52	10	1
Allocations of space within the hospital	2	41	14	2
Bed allocations by service*	5	36	13	3
How house staff members are paid	7	33	11	4
Personnel policies and procedures	16	25	8	7
Determining who is appointed, and with what privileges, to the medical staff*	18	12	7	13

*These are patient care decisions.

the hospital is more strongly in the hands of the medical school and its clinical faculty than management of the support services is in the hands of hospital administration.

In drawing a distinction between governance and operating decisions, the distribution of influence between board level and administration level, shown in tables 11.2 and 11.3, is quite sharp. As indicated in chapter 3, much of this power is concentrated at the university trustee level, and not the hospital board level.

In the past half-dozen years or so, a strong concern of hospital administrators has been to reduce or even eliminate control by the state government's bureaucracy over hospital operating decisions, and that remains today an important interest for a number of university hospitals. There is some justification for this interest. Simple correlations between state power and viability ($r = -.595$) and between state power and efficiency ($r = -.146$) indicate that a high level of state

Table 11.4 Simple Correlations of the Power of Key Groups in the Ownership Environment with UH Viability and Efficiency

	Viability		Efficiency	
	Correlation	Level of Significance	Correlation	Level of Significance
State power	−.595	.000	−.146	.30
Trustee power	−.197	.18	+.066	.64
University administration power	−.106	.47	−.172	.23
Medical school power	−.273	.06	−.361	.01
Hospital board power	+.273	.06	+.145	.31
Clinical chief involvement	+.131	.37	+.218	.12

influence on hospital operations is unlikely to serve the hospital well. As noted in chapter 3, the measure of viability does not measure the hospital's effectiveness in attracting state appropriations. When the viability measure includes state appropriations, the strong negative correlation with state power goes to zero ($r = .063$). Yet this statistic is itself interesting. Strong state influence, even with the appropriations that go with it, is not associated with higher levels of university hospital viability.

In states where the state bureaucratic control of the university is strong, an important strategy has been to grant the hospital greater autonomy from the university, and in this way solve the state control problem. Florida has been successful in this; Maryland and others are clearly moving in this direction. As noted in chapter 3, an indication of this movement is the relative youth of many hospitals' governing boards. The cooperation of the university, the medical school, and hospital administration in solving the state bureaucratic control problem is notable in several of the hospitals we studied.

In states where control by the state bureaucracy has not been an issue, some hospital administrators have nevertheless expressed an interest in greater autonomy from the university. Again, there is some support in the data for this. Table 11.4 shows the simple correlations between the power of key groups and the two measures of performance, viability and efficiency. One should not make too much of these figures, for in most cases the correlations are likely to contain influences not controlled for. Yet the generally negative relation between trustee, university administration, and medical school power with performance is clear. The power vested in key groups most distinct from the hospital board level tends to be the most negative in its impact on hospital viability. To put it more bluntly, those who don't know much about hospital issues tend to make the worst decisions.

To some university regents, presidents, vice-presidents, and medical school deans, the hospital administrators' quest for autonomy has appeared as distressing evidence that administrators have a knack for wrestling with the wrong problems, or worse, that they are disloyal to the ideals and interests of the university. To put it plainly, they are either fools or knaves [7]. Our study has convinced us there is a third possible explanation; it stems from hospital administration's professional interest in keeping the organization a fit instrument for delivering health care when the market environment is making this more difficult to do.

Some university hospitals are both viable and efficient, and we have explained this in earlier chapters in terms of a set of favorable environmental conditions. A supplementary explanation lies in the character of management and governance itself.

An issue of central interest is the form of governance, whether governance functions are located in either an academic health center board or a hospital board. A second variable of interest is the character of board orientation, whether to external threats and opportunities, or to internal management issues. A third variable of interest is power, the degree to which the hospital's board and administration together exercise significant influence on key policy and operating decisions. The fourth variable is the orientation of management toward external issues. Table 11.5 shows the simple correlations of these descriptors of hospital management and governance with efficiency. The correlations are not strong, though all are positive.

One can often gain a clearer understanding of relations between a set of possible influencing factors and an outcome by looking at the relations simultaneously. These partial correlations with efficiency are shown in table 11.6. The total correlation is shown at the bottom of the table.

As is evident in the table, 22 percent of the observed variation in efficiency can be explained by these variables, much of it by form of governance (AHC/hospital board) and by the orientation of hospital management. There is a basis here for saying that these management governance variables must be considered in explaining hospital efficiency.

The analysis in table 11.6 omits any consideration of environmen-

Table 11.5 Correlation of Governance and Management Variables with Hospital Viability and Efficiency

	Correlation with Viability	Correlation with Efficiency
AHC/hospital board	.229	.268
Board external orientation	.248	.107
HA/board power	.309	.091
External management orientation	.114	.260

Table 11.6 Multiple Correlation of Management and Governance Variables with Efficiency*

	Partial Correlation
AHC/hospital board	.292
External board orientation	.144
HA/board power	.096
External management orientation	.320

*Multiple correlation = .469; R^2 = .220.

tal impacts, and we have shown in earlier chapters that these are important explainers of hospital performance. Table 11.7 repeats the analysis, but with the environmental variable, "state pays welfare" added to the list. Holding the effect of this variable constant tends to reduce the partial correlations of the management and governance variables. It is generally true (with an exception we shall note shortly) that environmental and internal management and governance variables act consistently in their effect on performance. That is, high values of a variable such as "state pays welfare," that are directly associated with improved performance, are also associated with high values of management and governance variables such as "external management orientation" that correlate with improved performance.

It is particularly true that ownership-environment variables associated with low performance are also associated with low values of the management and governance variables. That is, appropriate structures for a strong and externally oriented hospital governance and management are harder to establish in a setting in which the hospital is protected by substantial state or university financial support and supervision. Perhaps this can be seen most clearly in the negative

Table 11.7 Multiple Correlation with Efficiency (Including State Pays Welfare)*

	Partial Correlation
AHC/hospital board	.239
External board orientation	.015
HA/board power	.128
External management orientation	.314
State pays welfare	.275

*Multiple correlation = .528; R^2 = .279.

Table 11.8 Correlations of Management and Governance Variables with State Appropriations

Variable	Correlation
AHC/hospital board	−.222
HA/board power	−.290
External management orientation	−.092
Board external orientation	−.377

relation that each of them has in the amount of state appropriation. Table 11.8 shows each of these correlations.

An important qualification needs to be made to this analysis. Appropriations and other forms of state support are the survival margin for many university hospitals. It is well to remember that the actual values of the viability index (which shows net surplus less appropriation) are uniformly negative for state university hospitals. In hospitals with high levels of state appropriations, these negative values are very large. If efforts to strengthen management and governance in these university hospitals lessen the certainty of receiving state support, such efforts may not serve the hospital well. These are truly "appropriations-dependent" hospitals. State support may take forms other than direct state appropriations, as Schramm has described, and suggests to us the wisdom of university hospitals giving up some discretion in return for ". . . predictable changes and sheltering from uncompensated care" [8].

It is possible for university hospitals to have both strong management and governance, and a protected environment, but this is less common than having strong leadership in an unprotected environment. Interestingly, the worst case for performance is to have high protection and low leadership power. One can almost say that in order to have efficiency and intrinsic viability, university hospitals need strong management and governance to protect them from their protectors! Table 11.8 has already shown that strong leadership and an external orientation is less likely with high appropriations than with low; this suggests a significant role for strong management and governance in just the settings where it is most difficult to develop such strength.

Marshall Meyer, in an extensive study of finance departments in local governments, concluded that weak leadership of a department permitted changes in the department's environment to have strong effects on the department's operation [9]. Strong leadership muted these effects. Our data seem to parallel those of Meyer. When a hospital has strong leadership, it is able to marshal the resources to anticipate and adapt to (ownership) environment challenges, and to initiate the actions necessary to protect the viability of the university hospital. This line of reasoning would suggest that the ownership environment presents the fundamental challenge to university hospitals; as this challenge diminishes, the attention of all shifts to the competitive environment.

Effect of Competition Pressure on Governance

It will be useful to return to one of the path diagrams used in chapter 7 in order that the data discussed here may be linked to those findings (figure 11.1 is the same as figure 7.2).

Three "paths" are of particular interest, and are circled on the figure. They show the by-now-familiar conclusions that competition tends to support performance, and state appropriation tends not to support it. But competition has no indirect effect when operating through the management-orientation variable, where one might expect it to be strongest. At least the awareness of competition by hospital management would seem to be a necessity in order to have high levels of competition cause efficiency. Quite possibly the effect of heightened competition, at least for some period, is to heighten the concern of the university administration, and to cause some increase in supervision of university operations and attention to them. Paradoxically, the market pressures that require stronger governance and management work in parallel with the ownership pressures that help to weaken them. Presumably two forces are at work. One is a tendency toward resolving hospital problems at higher levels so that decisions will be made with state, university, medical school, or clinical faculty interests foremost [10]. The second is a tendency toward separating out

Figure 11.1 Impact of Environment, Governance and Management on Efficiency ($N = 34$*)

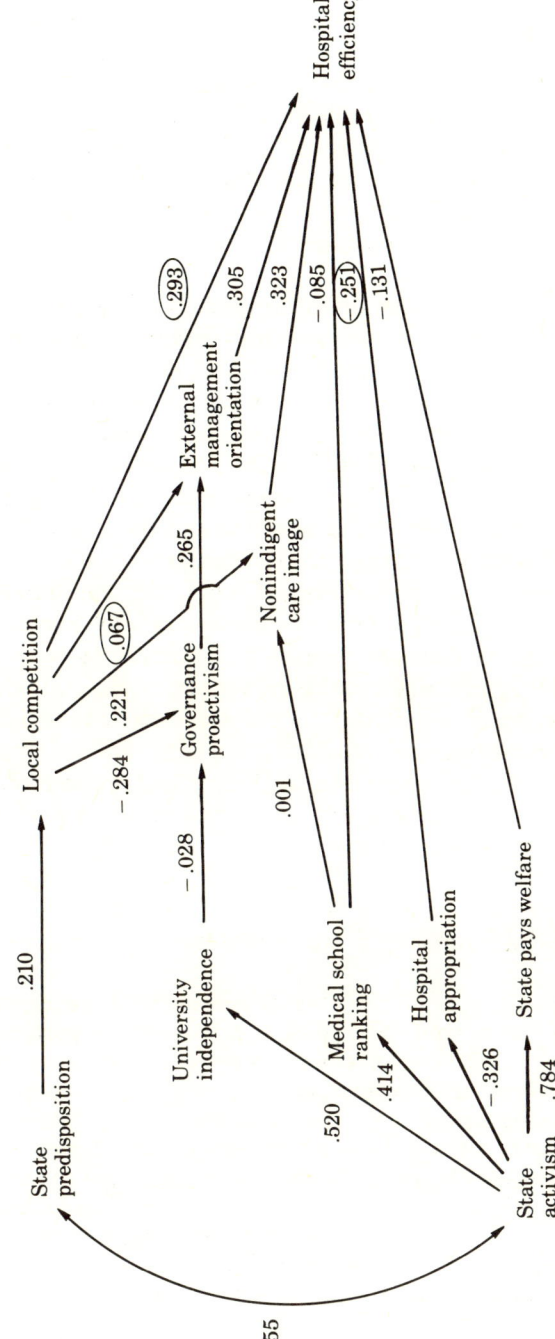

Reprinted with permission from *Medical Care* 23(July 1985):859.
*All coefficients are expected to be generalizable to the population of state university hospitals because sample N approximates population.
†Variance explained = 37 percent.

related problem sets, such as those of the university hospital, and developing structures to deal with them individually [11]. Both pressures have been relatively steady over the years, and their inconsistent demands help explain the character of university hospitals. As the competition and regulatory environment has become more complicated and less benign, both pressures are accentuated, and the inconsistent demands are frustrating the efforts of university hospital directors to make the hospital a fit instrument for achieving a viable set of outcomes.

We had expected that increased competition would increase the influence of management. That is, we assumed that the greater urgency of the problems would cause the problem-solving capacity to be concentrated where those problems could best be handled. This has not been the case. Perhaps we should have assumed just the opposite, that the study would not have been supported by the hospitals unless we found just what we did! What causes this perverse relation between the need for problem-solving capacity in the hospital and the low influence of hospital management? We suggest three possibilities below.

Possibility one: it is not perverse. When things become difficult for the hospital, then the university system as a whole should be kept centralized, moving the decision-making power from the hospital further up the hierarchy in the AHC, the university, or the state, in order to prevent short-sighted decisions. It would appear that this is happening in some universities, and may be seen as a shift of university administration energy toward addressing the management problems of the hospital. It is well to remember that a university hospital in trouble can present the medical school, and the university, with serious problems.

Possibility two: the relation is perverse, and intendedly so. One university hospital administrator put it this way:

> I believe that some states do not want the hospital to be operated too well, because they do not want their political constituencies, particularly in the case of legislators and governors, to perceive that too much of the public largess is going into operation of a "poor peoples' hospital." Also, I believe sometimes universities do not want the hospitals or the academic medical centers to get "too big for their britches," overshadow the university or to overshadow other important components of the university. . . . There are . . . other motives for not wanting the hospital to operate too successfully, but this really is a fundamental factor; it may be that we CEOs . . . are hired to do a fair job, but not too good a job and no one ever tells us that, but that really is the case and it takes a long time to find that out.

This point of view will sound absurd to some, but we believe there are many university hospital directors in the country to whom it would not sound absurd. Yet that does not make it true. There is also a third explanation.

Possibility three: the relation is perverse, but not intended. State, university, medical school, and clinical faculty interests are valid and legitimate ones, and they necessarily shape the thinking and orientation of those who direct these entities. Thus, for example, the establishment of an HMO is considered against criteria that measure its impact on the clinical services, on the teaching function, on subspecialist referral networks, on university good will, possible complaints from the legislature, and so on. No one is carefully calculating how to keep the university hospital doing just well enough but not too well. Rather, they are calculating how to protect and serve the legitimate interests they represent. They do not see a growing threat to the university hospital—only the growing threat to their own valid and legitimate interests. Hospital administrators are concerned with the bottom line, and rightfully so. The clinical faculty are understandably more concerned with teaching and research.

The difference between the second and third possibility is very large. If those in the ownership environment want the hospital just barely to survive, then conflict is inevitable and strategies (by both parties) need to be selected with eventual victory in mind. However, if those in the ownership environment do not recognize the consequences of allowing governance and management decisions to be made with inadequate understanding of the hospital's interests, then a strategy aimed at building structures that can both recognize and resolve differing interests is appropriate. Our data do not suggest universities are doomed to fail that strengthen management capacity at the university level rather than the hospital level. Instead the evidence suggests that up to the present time this strategy has not hurt hospital viability in the most competitive and least protected settings. The data do show that hospitals in these settings are twice as likely to have strong management and governance, and one may speculate that in the post-DRG era this proportion may have to grow.

We must not lose sight of the fact that we are here discussing differences among university hospitals, and concentrating for the moment on hospitals at the high end of the competitive spectrum. It is the recent intensification of competitive pressure that is forcing attention to where power resides for operating decisions and governance policymaking. It is also clear why the expectation of great competitive pressure in the future is so worrisome to university hospital CEOs.

Shifts in the locus of power have been taking place, and certain patterns of organizational adaptation are reasonably clear. Four of these are described below.

Strong AHC Administration

Historically, the responsibility for integrating the multiple missions of teaching, research, and patient care resided with the medical school administration, and included in that office a subordinate position usually called a hospital administrator. It often worked well. The modern-day equivalent is to retitle the medical school dean as the vice-president for health affairs (VPHA) or chancellor of the medical campus, and to give that person three or four key subordinates, each appropriately titled: one for medical school teaching and research, one for clinical affairs, perhaps one for financial affairs, and one for hospital administration. In some places it still works well.

Strong University Administration

It is fair to note that three of the four subordinates described above are likely to spend most of their time and energy on issues common to all tertiary-care facilities. Perhaps because of this, the second structural solution is to let the dean remain a dean, and then cut the hospital administrator tie to the medical school and switch it to university administration so that the growing financial, legal, personnel, purchasing, public relations, and other interdependencies can (from the university's perspective) be managed more effectively. Patient care remains with the dean, though the significant direct linkages to the university often make this an uneasy relationship. The mediator between the medical school and hospital on patient care issues, often titled Chief of Staff, has a difficult and sensitive role, and the clinical chiefs frequently discover room for maneuver in such a structure, and even more room for complaints. Sometimes a new official, also called VPHA or chancellor of the medical campus, is given the charge of helping these groups work together. (But this is a very different role from the VPHA described above.) We know of one place where this has worked well; it is possible there are others, but in essence it complicates the management problem without solving the governance problem.

Strong Hospital Administration

A third structural solution is best seen as shifting the responsibility for resolving the conflict of different interests to hospital administration. In this model not only support services but financial affairs is the domain of hospital administration, and the chief of staff's primary allegiance shifts from the medical school to the hospital. This model, even more than the first, requires a brilliant leader, for it is extremely difficult for academics and those who manage the academic enterprise to subordinate themselves to a service function in a university.

Separate Hospital Governance

The difficulty noted above is what gives central importance to the fourth model, the third model sans brilliant leader but with an effective hospital board. (It sharply reduces the need for a "great leader" as hospital director.) This model is new to state universities, somewhat more common among the privates, and is of course the closest to those universities such as Harvard and Johns Hopkins which do not own hospitals at all. Its actual success is blurred by the larger number of universities which have put in place bodies called hospital boards that are largely figureheads; real governance has continued to take place elsewhere.

Our own reading of the current environment is that either the first or fourth model will be the most effective, and the most feasible. The advantage of the first (strong AHC administration) is that it facilitates the use of conventional and well-understood bureaucratic controls to achieve a balance between teaching, research, and patient care, and to secure coordination between the hospital and medical staff-clinical faculty. The advantage of the fourth model (separate hospital governance) is that it provides separate forums for addressing the complex issues now facing university hospitals, as well as the equally difficult issues facing schools of medicine and the other health professions. We believe this fourth model is somewhat more flexible and easily adapted to changing power distributions among the key groups described at the beginning of this chapter. But it reduces the capacity of the state, the university, or the medical school to exercise control through conventional lines of bureaucratic authority, and perhaps for this reason may be resisted by these groups.

In situations where the university hospital lacks intrinsic viability, the second model (strong university administration) may be preferred, simply because it is the one most suited to maintaining significant state support for the hospital. However we are less optimistic than Schramm that such state support can be sustained, much less increased. For the short term, many university hospitals must act in order to protect their state support. We believe, however, that they are unwise to depend on it as a permanent substitute for intrinsic viability.

REFERENCES

1. Munson, E., and A. McCulloch. The university-owned hospital: Pterodactyl or phoenix? Paper presented at University Hospital Ad Hoc Study Group, Phoenix, Arizona, January 21, 1980.
2. Allison, R., and J. Dalston. Governance of university-owned teaching hospitals. *Inquiry* 19(1982)3–17.
3. Munson, E., and A. McCulloch, University hospital.
4. Hogness, J. The complex relationships of academic health centers. In *Proceedings of the 1976 annual meeting of the association for academic health centers.* Washington, D.C.: Association for Academic Health Centers, 1976.
5. Westerman, J. A requiem for the university hospital. *Health Care Management Review* 5(Spring 1980):17–24.
6. Petersdorf, R., and M. Wilson. The four horsemen of the apocalypse: Study of academic medical center governance. *Journal of the American Medical Association* 247(1982):1153–61.
7. Westerman, Requiem, p. 23.
8. Schramm, C. The teaching hospital and the future role of state government. *New England Journal of Medicine* 308(1983):41–45.
9. Meyer, M.W. Leadership and organizational structure. In *Environments and Organizations,* edited by M.W. Meyer. San Francisco: Jossey-Bass Publishers, 1978, pp. 212–23, 229.
10. Ebert, R., and S. Brown. Academic health centers. *New England Journal of Medicine* 308(1983):1200–1208.
11. Wilson, M., R. Knapp, and A. Jones. The growing managerial imperative of the academic medical center. In *Health Management for Tomorrow* edited by S. Levy and T. McCarthy. Philadelphia: J.B. Lippincott Co., 1980, pp. 81–108.

TWELVE

Conclusions

In this final chapter we record the more significant observations and conclusions we have reached as a result of doing the study, and end with some brief speculations about the future for university hospitals.

THE CENTRALITY OF THE OWNERSHIP ENVIRONMENT

The market environment is getting worse, and the control structure of many university hospitals is ill-equipped to meet the challenge they face. Contingency theory suggests, and our data confirm, that structure provides programmed solutions to routine demands or problems in the provision of health care. Because we are dealing with institutions that produce essentially the same services, their structures differ primarily in response to differences in the nonroutine demands presented by their environments. Consequently, the question becomes, "What structures work best in different types of environments?" Our major task, therefore, has been to specify what we mean by environment, and to develop types and measures of environments.

One of us has observed elsewhere that

> university hospitals have to contend with two external environments: the internal environment of the university and the elements outside the control of both the university and the hospital. . . . Rather than serve the hospital, the university board is often a part of the environment that the hospital must somehow adapt to or try to influence. [1]

Being relevant to the hospital but beyond its control, and by orientation often more a source of constraints than support, owners are frequently more correctly classified as part of the hospital's "environment" than merely another level within the hospital's bureaucratic hierarchy.

In our field studies we observed that not all universities constrain their hospitals; generally, private universities are more supportive and less constraining. Hence we thought initially that ownership per se is a primary causal variable identifying supportive owners. However, further research showed that some state-owned universities are not supportive of their hospitals. The political culture of the state is the important underlying variable that determines whether a state supports its state-owned university hospital. In essence, states having a highly progressive or proactive political culture treat their university and its hospital much as private universities treat their hospitals.

The key is the function served by their hospitals. Private university-owned hospitals must be self-supporting, for they are too expensive for private universities to subsidize. When their medical schools are research-oriented, their control of an independent stream of research funds gives them greater independence from their parent university. In like manner, in politically progressive states the state makes separate provisions for indigent medical care—through Medicaid in hospitals all over the state, and through city and county hospitals. As a result, the university hospital is not expected to be an indigent care center, and the state does not subsidize it as such. This nondependence or low dependence on state appropriation means that little or no state funds are flowing through the university and thereby giving state and university officials financial leverage to control the hospital. Because both the state and university services are almost always organized functionally, this means: (1) various functional parts of the hospital are not controlled by remote officials and by criteria foreign to hospital goals; (2) there is less tendency to centralize power—which is the inherent tendency of any functional structure. Not only is the hospital thus spared these bureaucratic controls and tendency to overcentralization, it is also free to be more attuned to the needs of the medical staff. In these same states, medical schools are typically more research oriented—as are their universities. Research funds give both the university and the medical school greater autonomy. Research by the medical faculty means that the medical staff of the university hospital refers patients there for medical rather than financial reasons. Consequently, the hospital becomes more competitive and tertiary-care oriented. In summary, state-owned university hospitals in politically proactive or progressive states have goals and structures quite similar to private hospitals.

Our findings indicate that private hospitals and publicly owned hospitals in politically progressive states have performed better than public hospitals in politically conservative states. The question then becomes, "How do the control structures of the latter differ from those of the former?" Operationally, appropriation is the ownership element that distinguishes among those that tend toward support and those that tend toward constraint. Because most private university-owned hospitals receive no appropriation, we will focus primarily here on public hospitals—in this case, contrasting them on the basis of the level of state appropriation.

Appropriation-Dependent Hospitals

As we have shown in our analysis, the control of public hospitals receiving proportionately large appropriation (relative to their total revenues) varies greatly from those receiving little or no appropriation. State university hospitals receiving proportionately large appropriations have less influential governing boards and management, *and lower performance,* than those receiving little or no appropriations. Yet in either case the more influential boards and management contribute strongly to improved performance.

We believe that the explanation of this phenomenon lies in the importance of avoiding a diffusion of power in such settings. Appropriations flow downward from the state and the university through functional organization structures, and each functional official is thereby given some leverage to use in exacting controls over his or her function as it occurs within the university hospital. When hospital functions are influenced by remote officials at several levels removed from the hospital, the hospital is unable to respond to its competitive market environment. The resulting structure tends to be diffuse rather than coordinated. What typical hospital administrator in this type of hospital has not bemoaned civil service regulations that keep the salaries of the nursing staff below what is required to attract nurses in the hospital's labor market? What is needed is a personnel system coordinated with the production (patient care) system. Unfortunately, this lateral coordination among hospital functions is precisely that which the structure of the state and university are ill-prepared to provide. If university vice-presidents think of integrating their functions with others, they do so for the good of the university, not for the good of one division of the university. This is the classic predicament of a product-type division embedded within a functionally structured, larger organization. University hospitals are in that predicament.

Some public hospitals do provide a generous appropriation without insisting on large controls, and the results seem to favor all parties concerned. It is against administrative nature for this to occur, but it does occur, and the officials involved are almost legends in the field. (To call them lucky would be unfair, for these officials may have been the ones responsible for their state governments and universities providing unencumbered funding.) What we are saying is this: a state can provide appropriations and ensure their proper stewardship through strong leadership, perhaps primarily outside of normal bureaucratic channels. The issue here is a focus of control, more than the level at which it is exercised. A hospital must be coordinated by a body or small set of officials who see its interests clearly and who orient it toward its most critical environments. It requires focused leadership, not a diffuse and shifting distribution of power. Although it is true that this focus is better provided close to the hospital (i.e., decentralized), the greater requirement is to have influence concentrated at some level. Not surprisingly, for university hospitals with high dependence on state appropriations it may be more political to have this influence at high levels, close to the state, than at low levels, close to the production of health care. Hence, although important considerations for success include how many are involved in governance and at what level in the hierarchy, of the two, "how many" is the greater consideration for this type of hospital. These hospitals require focused leadership.

Appropriation-Independent Hospitals

State university hospitals receiving little or no appropriations have more influential governing boards and management and *better performance* than those receiving large appropriations. Yet within this subset of hospitals the more influential boards and management contribute little to improve performance.

We believe the explanation of this phenomenon lies in the importance of decentralization. As the importance of protecting state appropriations decreases, the importance of market responsiveness increases, and the problem focus shifts from the university-state relationship to the medical school–hospital relationship. Structures that effectively resolve conflicts between the goals of patient care, teaching, and research take on added significance. The importance of a strong board and management is clear, but the vital margin is provided by structures that deal effectively with patient-care management decisions. Diffusion of power remains a problem, but is overshadowed by the importance of giving power to those closest to the production process —that is, hospital administration and the clinical faculty. The relevant part of the ownership environment is now contained within the university, and from the hospital perspective the critical problem is building a capacity to respond rapidly to market demands.

We have written the preceding—as if there were two distinct types of university hospitals—in order to sharpen the contrast between the two settings. Of course there is a continuum, not a dichotomy. Perhaps the simplest summary is the following: university hospitals with high dependence on the state need most to collect power; those with high dependence on their own resources need most to decentralize it.

THE CHANGING CHARACTER OF COMPETITION

Even before the advent of DRGs, the reorganization of some university hospitals for the purpose of efficiency and viability made eminent sense. The DRGs, while viewed by many hospitals as confining and limiting their discretion, may in fact support alterations in the current pattern of relationships between health organizations. The potential changes to be induced by the DRG system may in fact facilitate the provision of advanced tertiary care. Since such a level of care is not usually routine and since there are usually not enough patients to create an economy of scale for many nonuniversity hospitals, it would make financial sense to refer some patients to the university hospital.

This scenario is still to evolve, if indeed it does. But it illustrates that regardless of how the market shifts, the fortunes of the university hospital are subject to the vicissitudes of a larger environmental context made up of other health delivery organizations. The advantages of the university hospital are greatly enhanced, of course, if it becomes a more integral part of the health care network in its service area. Many external interviewees lamented the historical position of "splendid isolation" maintained by some university hospitals. It has not helped the university hospital to be so inward looking. It has been helped by the external orientation of management, spending time with legislation, regulatory agencies, reimbursers, and other providers in the service area.

The impact of changing payment systems will be felt inside the hospital as well. DRGs can also illustrate this truth. Under such a payment system, documented use of hospital resources will have to be DRG-specific, and this opens the way to identify all the more clearly the profitable and unprofitable service activities in the hospital. Cross-service subsidization will be increasingly difficult to conceal. Internal strife may result between colleagues in different service areas, and CEOs may find themselves in a totally new "ballgame."

From the CEO perspective, starting afresh has a certain appeal. It may mean starting the university hospital afresh as a new corporation separate from the university system. We have shown in chapter 7 that the influence of the state on the university hospital is mediated through the university processes. The inertia this adds to that already produced by the large university system and the concomitant lack of decision-making latitude on the part of the university hospital administrator makes a separate corporation appear administratively attractive to hospital personnel. It can then deal directly with the state legislature, negotiate with legitimate authority with the medical school, and deal with tax and capital related matters separately from the university. The fact that some university hospitals have successfully incorporated in this way makes the alternative appear all the more attractive.

Separate incorporation is a double-edged sword. Two parties are at risk: the hospital itself, and the university. A profitable hospital is not an institution that the parent university will wish to let go. Conversely, a money-losing hospital is less anxious to separate from the parent university. Of course in some settings the marriage between hospital and university remains healthy and robust; corporate restructuring is not the panacea for all university hospitals. However, when a hospital is confronted with structurally enforced inertia internally and increasing competition externally, corporate restructuring makes sense.

A current compromise of having separate hospital boards in some universities may be a sufficient stop-gap measure if those boards can really act with authority. It is unclear that all of those boards do. In the absence of such authority, failures of the university hospital may find new or additional scapegoats.

The uncertainty looming on the horizon is, as usual, the prospective-payment system. If the university hospital can benefit from this, then the survival issue is at least temporarily resolved and the need to restructure corporately is reduced. If, on the other hand, DRGs turn out to erode the viability of university hospitals, then a drastic policy must be considered for the survival of some university hospitals.

THE ROLE OF HOSPITAL GOVERNANCE

The governance function for a university hospital is not yet a well-accepted notion in all universities; one does not speak of "governance" of the book store, grounds and maintenance, or the dormitories. For some in the university, its hospital is simply one of the services necessary to the teaching and research enterprise. This attitude is much less common than it was a decade ago, but the specific role of hospital governance still varies widely between different universities. This has permitted us to make judgments about the causes and consequences of these variations.

Weak Hospital Governance and Weak Hospital Management Go Together

This relation is apparent when one considers the management problems of support services, finance, and patient care.

For a number of hospitals, the development of good management is hindered by state and university involvement in the management of support services. The problem for the hospital is more one of mixed control than absence of control, or most directly, a control that is not responsive to the legitimate needs of the hospital. Quite a number of hospital directors see greater hospital autonomy as a way to escape from these problems. An equally reasonable approach, and one more feasible in some places, is to organize power sufficient to focus attention on support service issues. With few exceptions they are simply the result of bad management practices at state, university or hospital levels.

Yet, fundamentally, it is absurd that managing support services should be a concern of top management at all. Where else can you find a $100 million annual operation in which problems of repairing windows or changing pay grades requires attention at the top management level? And find such hospitals not once, but repeatedly? Unfortunately, solving the problem of support services will not solve the problem of governance, as a number of university hospitals know.

The diminution of federal research and education funds, the tightening of reimbursement rules, the gradual loss of state appropriations, and the competition for patients threatens to change the university hospital from a net exporter to a net importer of funds from the university. To respond to these threats creatively requires actions that focus on the situation of the hospital, not that of the university. A possible strategy is for university financial officers to become knowledgeable, skillful, and dedicated hospital financial officers. Alternatively, the university may choose instead to shift responsibility for financial management decisions to the hospital or the academic health center. In other words, the university either can risk having hospital needs dominate its attention and energy, or it can let the university hospital loose. Neither is an attractive solution, and if the university hospital is heavily dependent on state appropriations, the second option may be most unattractive to the hospital. Probably very few university hospitals that depend heavily on the state for financial support can be disengaged effectively from the university. The increased uncertainty for both the hospital and the university would be substantial, and the possibility of competition for state funds undesirable to both.

So for some university hospitals, significantly increased autonomy is out of the question so long as they depend on state appropriations not explicitly linked to the cost of providing indigent care. For the other hospitals—the growing number that depend almost entirely on patient revenues—the finance problem is really the support service problem writ large. The university and the medical school must be convinced that a strong hospital will serve their long-term interests. A facility that can be constantly tapped into by many groups will, in the end, serve neither them nor the patients very well. Quite a few university hospitals are wrestling with governance at this level. Sometimes the solution is to increase the hospital's financial autonomy from the university and medical school; sometimes it is to increase the financial autonomy of the academic health center as a whole. The tactic of forming an academic health center that retains university control of hospital finance is, of course, little more than redrawing lines to accommodate one more coordinator, and is in our view dysfunctional.

Yet even when key hospital financial decisions are being made with the hospital's interest in mind, the problem is not solved. There remains the problem of making patient-care policy decisions for patients and the community, not for medical students or faculty research. No university hospital wants such decisions to ignore teaching and research, because all university hospitals depend on the clinical faculty and the residents to differentiate their product. But university hospitals increasingly want patient and community health-care needs to dominate the decision criteria when hospital resources are being allocated. Cecil Sheps has used the metaphor of a married couple: they both need each other, but find the relationship works best when each is able, with equal strength, to negotiate with and accommodate the other. As we have said, some hospital–medical school relationships work well with the medical school dominating the relationship. But we believe the tide is running against this form of relationship, and that in a university setting critical patient-care policy decisions are going to have to be made by a governing body capable of making them stick, if management of patient care is to be effective.

A Board Is a Good Place in Which to Concentrate the Hospital Governance Function

A board is not the only place in which to concentrate hospital governance, and a satisfactory substitute is to have a strong and effective individual in the academic health center vice-president position, or in the university president position. Such an individual could also operate from the medical-school dean position or even that of the hospital director. Such individuals are not all-powerful but they are unusually skillful in building strength and securing support from inside and outside the university. Nevertheless there are reasons why hospital boards are a good place to concentrate the governance function:

— It is organizationally easier to build a good board than to find a brilliant leader.
— In a board the onus of an unpopular decision is on no one person. In a difficult and changing environment, such decisions need to be made more often. "Depersonalizing" such decisions is one of the strengths of the board form of governance.
— Board membership can accommodate diverse perspectives, and change to reflect new perspectives that must or should be considered when fundamental issues are crystallized into governance questions.

It Is Better to Have a Strong Board Than a Representative One

In a sense this is a depressing conclusion: it argues for doing well what you want to do, rather than trying harder for what you ought to do. The reason that makes this choice preferable is the importance of having a clear center of authority when there are multiple interests, and significant power to enforce them. We believe that the pressures from the environment will be responded to more effectively when there is a clear focus for crucial policy decisions. That is, a strong board will in the end try harder to do what they ought to do . . . or else.

Such a governing body must recognize the quality that differentiates the university hospitals from other teaching hospitals. In the university hospital, teaching is not an add-on to patient care, nor is research a device to increase tertiarity. Rather, each is an end in itself. The distinctive role of the university hospital is to provide a setting where the fundamental issues of defining health and effectively supporting it are addressed and resolved—not in the abstract, but in the concrete delivery of care to those who need it.

One may expect hospital management to understand the basic intertwining of these issues, but someone has to mind the store, run the hospital, and be concerned with the organization's financial viability. This viability rests on performance in the patient-care area, not in teaching or research. Someone has to be primarily concerned with making the hospital a fit instrument for providing patient care. Therefore, it is at the governance level that the difficult questions of meshing the three missions and defining the patient-care domain (what services to what groups of people in what geographic area) must be addressed.

Board Membership

The meshing of the three missions can be addressed by an outside board when traditions are so strong and values so widely shared that the interdependence with the university and medical school rests as firmly on beliefs as it does on logic. Johns Hopkins Hospital and Massachusetts General Hospital illustrate this reality. Yet it is reasonable to expect that the obligation to serve teaching and research goals will be more effectively met if some of the people deeply committed to the teaching and research enterprise are present on the board. Florida has followed this model in its hospital board, and hospitals with academic health center boards have addressed the issue by having governance responsible for the guidance of both the health schools and the hospital.

Multiple centers of power are characteristic of university hospitals; the control of key resources required for survival is widely scattered, and it is important to attract new resources (as in philanthropy or in the development and sale of new services). Among the most important of these power centers are the clinical chiefs. Their potential influence may arise from at least three sources: the substantial authority they have within their departments, the impressive effect clinical departments can have on patient revenues, and the fact that the integration of patient care, teaching, and research happens (or doesn't happen) at the clinical department level. Thus it is common for the clinical staff to be represented, often through one or more chiefs, on the hospital board. In more traditional boards of nonprofit institutions, this representation of groups that can benefit themselves is less common. There is genuine value in building a sense of trusteeship in the hospital or AHC board, and that mind- and value-set is more difficult to achieve when some board members can benefit themselves or their interests by the decisions taken by the board.

The same conflict between the board as trustee and the board as collector of power arises in using ex-officio members; that is, having a board made up of whoever is holding a specified office. Being selected to a board by virtue of an office held encourages a person to act as a representative of the interests of the office rather than as a trustee of the institution. A second disadvantage of ex-officio members is more prosaic; they simply change too often, and for reasons that may be unrelated to their potential for fulfilling the trusteeship role. Nevertheless the issue of who has power remains vital, and the conclusion we draw from the study is that it is more important to have a strong board than to have a representative one.

A University Board of Trustees Is Less Likely to Qualify as a Strong Board Than One Dedicated to the Hospital, or Academic Health Center

Of course university boards have power; legal ownership can be the basis of a great variety of successful coalitions. But they often do not have enough knowledge of hospital issues to make that power effective, or the time, energy, experience, or, most important, the interest to accumulate such knowledge.

Nevertheless, in circumstances where much of the policy making and conflict resolution is mediated by an individual of exceptional competence, it may well be preferable to have no intervening layer between the university governing body and such a person. Organizational amenities may require that one or more official positions appear on the organization chart between that person and the board, but we are speaking of the real relationships.

HOSPITAL BOARDS TAKE TIME TO BECOME EFFECTIVE

The experience of the hospitals interviewed in our field study is that the early months (or sometimes years) of a board's operation are characterized by one or more of the following:

- Figuring out what is their turf, and what belongs to some other group or body. The other group may be above, below, or beside them, and the uncertainty may be about issue areas (i.e., just how much is medical staffing or nurse staffing our concern?), or about the appropriate type of involvement in an area (i.e., do we rubber stamp a clinical chief appointment, or do we shape selection criteria?).
- Fighting fires and assisting management. Managers new to the experience of dealing with boards sometimes use them extensively as a sounding board and consultive group for difficult but essentially operational problems. Thus early activity of new boards is often focused on urgent and sometimes exciting but essentially ephemeral issues.
- Report receiving and proposal approving. The final-authority functions of the board are the simplest to activate, and also leave the most policy discretion in the hands of the administration. Movement to a flowing and probing discussion of issues at the point where the proper framing of the question is still unclear, and the appropriate criteria therefore undefined, is far more difficult to achieve and normally comes later (if at all) in the life of a board. But it also is the most effective point for a board to influence the direction of administrative action.

Board membership for anyone except insiders is a part-time activity, but for a board to be effective it must become a deliberative body. The functions of a board include a variety of activities, but among the most important is determining the direction of the institution: this is rarely done effectively by receiving recommendations and voting on them. Policies should instead develop from discussions, which lead in turn to requests for recommendations that shape planning premises. It is far more difficult to develop the culture of a deliberative body than the culture of a proposal-approving one. It is one of the reasons that large boards are forced to sacrifice the board as a whole to the proposal-approving function, and develop committees for the deliberative function. It is instructive that some university boards of trustees (the University of Michigan among them) refuse to use committees, in spite of the remarkable diversity of the enterprise they guide.

THE FUTURE

Predicting the future in a turbulent environment is futile, but in some respects the environment of university hospitals is less turbulent than it is fast-changing. What are some of the more predictable changes, and what consequences will they have for university hospitals?

1. Buyers of health care will continue to shop for better buys, while providers of health care will continue to experiment with innovative delivery systems that offer better care for less money. Patterns of usage of health care facilities will become increasingly unstable, and will penalize those providers that can neither protect their revenue sources nor adapt quickly enough to find new ones. With each passing year, more university hospitals and clinics will face the same competitive pressure some are facing today. The capacity to adapt and to develop and quickly implement new services will become progressively more important.

2. Short of a major economic boom, the federal government will continue to search for ways to constrain the cost increases in its major social programs, and will continue to experiment with new forms of regulation and more effective methods of locating and eliminating avoidable health care costs. Case-based payment systems provide an opportunity to drive payments down toward the level of the least-cost producer, and are also an effective method of squeezing educational and other subsidies out of the reimbursement system. The surplus of physicians will continue, providing a constant counter pressure—direct or indirect—on federal subsidies for medical education. Pure cost pressure on university hospitals will continue unabated.

3. Multiunit systems will continue to grow in size, in ability to attract capital, and in emphasis on penetrating markets and expanding market share.
   Increasingly, university hospitals will face aggressively managed systems that are both larger and better financed than the university hospital. Cooperation or competition with these units will be inescapable, both in serving a patient population and in providing an attractive setting for parts of the medical

school's clinical faculty to practice. University hospitals will continue to lose some of the advantage their comparatively large size has given them. Indeed, the higher cost per case associated with large unit size may cause them to retain all the economic disadvantages of large size, at the same time that they are losing the bargaining and prestige advantages that large size once brought them.

4. High-technology medicine will continue to grow in importance, and university hospitals will continue to have a strong comparative advantage over other hospitals in providing a site for the development and early implementation of new discoveries. The natural synergy between teaching and patient care will continue to protect their comparative advantage in providing highly intensive care, as well as highly innovative and complex care. The openness to new ideas and methods characteristic of universities should give them an advantage in developing new delivery systems as well, such as extensive use of nonphysician primary care providers—but it is unlikely to do so. The important organizational innovations of the near future (the next decade) will be cost-saving innovations: and these will threaten professional boundaries. Universities are the natural home of innovation, but also of the health professions. Tertiary care, not economy, will continue to be the strong suit of the university hospital.

5. The decline of the state as a significant actor in the health care scene has been arrested. The importance of state resources and state support to some university hospitals will grow in the coming decade. Some may find the state is the most important resource supplier to cultivate. Although proactivist states are generally those which, like the federal government, find themselves overcommitted to social programs, the sense of ownership in the state university hospital is present to some degree in all of them. Therefore the possibility exists of nurturing a sense of responsibility for the hospital. To university hospitals now receiving significant appropriations, this may be the key to survival. State appropriations to the hospital are the most visible but not the only important financial support. University hospital medical staffs are also medical school clinical faculties, and generous support of the medical school serves the hospital's interests. The ability of the hospital to nurture this sense of responsibility for the hospital and medical school at the state level—at the same time it develops an understanding

at that level of the need for substantial freedom from state controls—may be the key to competing effectively and gradually reducing hospital dependence on state financial support.

As one considers the sunlight and shadow in this picture of the state university hospital's future, the bright spots appear to come from the possibility of continued support from the state, and the innovative, high-intensity care made possible by the university connection. The two things that the state university hospital has going for it is that it is a *state* and a *university* hospital. The challenges it faces come from the market environment. Unfortunately the difficulty the hospital faces in meeting these challenges also arise from its ownership environment—that is, its state and university connections. At the end of our study we have reached the conclusion that the challenges the state university hospital faces will not be met unless a satisfactory governance mechanism is interposed between the hospital and its ownership environment. It must be successful in buffering the hospital from the extraneous demand of this environment, at the same time that it perpetuates those values giving the university hospital its unique advantage.

REFERENCE

1. Allison, R.F., and J. Dalston. Governance of university-owned teaching hospitals. *Inquiry 19(Spring 1982):3–17.*

APPENDIX A

A Survey of the Management and Governance of University-Owned Teaching Hospitals

208 / Appendix A

 UNIVERSITY OF MINNESOTA
TWIN CITIES

Center for Health Services Research
School of Public Health
420 Delaware Street SE, Box 729
Minneapolis, Minnesota 55455

(612) 376-1895

A SURVEY OF THE MANAGEMENT AND GOVERNANCE OF UNIVERSITY-OWNED TEACHING HOSPITALS

SPONSORED BY

THE CONSORTIUM FOR THE STUDY OF UNIVERSITY HOSPITALS (CSUH)

CSUH BOARD MEMBERS:

James E. Moon
University of Alabama Hospitals

Richard H. Trethaway
University of South Alabama
Medical Center Hospital

Carl Fischer
University Hospital (Arkansas)

Robert Dickler
University Hospital (Colorado)

John Ives (President, CSUH)
Shands Teaching Hospital and Clinics
(Florida)

Jack Hall
University Hospital (Kentucky)

Morton Rapaport, M.D.
University of Maryland Hospital

Janice B. Wyatt
University of Massachusetts
Hospital

Jeptha W. Dalston, Ph.D.
University of Michigan Hospitals

Donald Van Hulzen
University of Minnesota Hospitals
and Clinics

Robert J. Baker
University Hospital and Clinic
(Nebraska)

Myles P. Lash (President-elect, CSUH)
Medical College of Virginia Hospitals

Roy S. Rambeck
University of Washington Hospitals

HONORARY MEMBER:

John W. Westerman
Allegheny Health, Education and
Research Corporation

CSUH RESEARCH STEERING
COMMITTEE:

Donald B. Clapp, J.D.
Vice President for Administration
University of Kentucky

William B. Deal, M.D.
Dean of Medicine
University of Florida College
of Medicine

John Ives (President, CSUH)
Executive Vice President
Shands Teaching Hospital and Clinics
(Florida)

William N. Kelly, M.D.
Chairman, Department of Internal
Medicine
University of Michigan Medical School

Paul G. Quie, M.D.
Chief of Staff
University of Minnesota Hospitals
and Clinics

Neal A. Vanselow, M.D.
Chancellor and Vice President
University of Nebraska College of Medicine

COOPERATING RESEARCH INSTITUTIONS
AND RESEARCH TEAM:

University of Michigan and
University of Minnesota

Thomas Choi, Ph.D.

Fred Munson, Ph.D.

Robert Allison, Ph.D.

PLEASE RETURN THE COMPLETED QUESTIONNAIRE
IN THE STAMPED ENVELOPE PROVIDED, OR SEND
TO:

Thomas Choi, Ph.D.
Center for Health Services Research
University of Minnesota
420 Delaware Street SE, Box 729
Minneapolis, MN 55455

Hospital Setting and Governance Information

SETTING

1. How many years have you been the CEO of this university hospital? (Write in Please) _____ years

2. How many years have you worked for the university and/or university hospital? (Write in please) _____ years

3. Please check (on the left hand side) which schools are part of your health sciences:

    _____ A. School of Medicine _____
    _____ B. School of Dentistry _____
    _____ C. School of Nursing _____
    _____ D. School of Pharmacy _____
    _____ E. School of Public Health _____
    _____ F. School of Allied Health _____
    _____ G. School of Veterinary Medicine _____
    _____ F. Other _____

4. Place a check AFTER each of the schools above that is next to or a part of the hospital campus.

5. How close is the hospital to the main university campus?

    _____ A. On the same campus
    _____ B. Physically separated, in same city
    _____ C. Physically separated, in a different city

6. If on the same campus, do you share building(s) with the Medical School and/or other health sciences?

    _____ A. Yes
    _____ B. No

7. Which of the following best describes the working relationships among the schools (including the university hospital) in your health sciences center?

    _____ A. Consistent and close working relationship.
    _____ B. Periodically close working relationship, depending on issues.
    _____ C. Rarely work together or coordinate with each other.

8. There are many alliances and coalitions between hospital departments, medical school, subspecialties, etc. These alliances have impact on influencing decisions relating to the hospital. In general, how stable are these alliances?

    _____ A. Very unstable. Largely depends on the issues and resources involved.
    _____ B. Moderately unstable
    _____ C. Moderately stable
    _____ D. Very stable. The alliances almost never change.

9. Overall, how much agreement is there among personnel in the hospital setting in terms of:

	Very Strong Agreement	Strong Agreement	Strong Disagreement	Very Strong Disagreement	Not an Issue
A. Whether the hospital should be strictly tertiary care					
B. How much research emphasis there should be					
C. How much service emphasis there should be					
D. How much indigent care there should be					

210 / Appendix A

DISTRIBUTION OF INFLUENCE IN THE UNIVERSITY HOSPITAL SETTING

10. In the questions to follow, we want to know the amount of influence exercised by each of eight officials or official groups in making 12 key decisions. Because you may not have all eight of these officials or groups, and because their titles may vary from those used on other campuses, we define each of them here.

KEY GROUPS (Definitions):

1. State: Elected or appointed officials employed by the state who are in any way involved in influencing the activities and funding of this state-owned hospital. (Excludes regulatory and rate-setting activities affecting all hospitals in state.)

2. Trustees or Regents: Formal body having final authority over this university or group of universities including yours, and typically comprised of non-employees of the state or university.

3. Hospital Board: Formal body, which may be a subset or committee of the Trustees, which has governance authority to address strategic, long-range policy matters for this hospital.

4. University Officials: High university officials and groups (president, vice presidents, etc.) excluding V.P. for the Health Sciences or Medical Center, if one exists.

5. Vice President for Health Sciences or Medical Center. (If this individual is also the Dean of the Medical School, check ☑ below and leave the VP/HS column blank in the questions to follow.)

IMPORTANT ☐ The VP/HS is also Dean of Medicine.

6. Medical School Administration: Dean and Associate Deans.

7. Clinical Chiefs: Medical School Department Chairman in their hospital roles as Chiefs of their respective clinical services.

8. Hospital Administration: Director and top hospital managers.

NOTE: If, for example, the Dean and Hospital Director are also on the hospital's board, you may wonder how you rate their influence as board members and in their respective executive positions. We do want you to separate these two forms or avenues of influence. Think of it this way: if groups are influential on a decision only insofar as they can influence the whole hospital board, the hospital board is highly influential. If a group on the hospital board can and does dictate, veto, or ignore hospital board actions, the hospital board is not influential.

Appendix A / 211

INSTRUCTIONS

Use the numbers (0 through 3) from the Scale of Influence to indicate the amount of influence exercised by each of the Key Groups for each of the 12 Key Decisions listed below:

SCALE OF INFLUENCE

3 = Major, decisive influence in shaping or determining the outcome.
2 = Substantial influence in shaping or determining the outcome
1 = Some influence in shaping or determining the outcome.
0 = Minor or no influence in shaping or determining the outcome.

IMPORTANT ⇨ KEY GROUPS (Refer to definitions on opposite page)

KEY DECISIONS	1. STATE	2. TRUSTEES	3. HOSPITAL BOARD	4. UNIV. OFFICIALS	5. V.P. FOR HEALTH	6. MED. SCHOOL ADMINISTRATION	7. CLINICAL CHIEFS	8. HOSPITAL ADMINISTRATION
1. Choose and/or appoint a new hospital CEO								
2. Reorganization at the governance level to give substantial autonomy to the university hospital								
3. Reorganization of hospital management (e.g., decentralization) to place accountability with second level managers.								
4. Expanding or contracting scope of medical services (e.g. trauma center)								
5. Allocations of space within the hospital								
6. Future directions, and emphasis on, clinical research								
7. Fund-raising (philanthropic)								
8. Personnel policies and procedures								
9. Operating budget allocations								
10. Decisions on capital budget allocations								
11. Decisions on amount and sources of capital financing (e.g. borrowing)								
12. Determining who is appointed, and with what privileges, to the medical staff								
13. How house staff members are paid								
14. Bed allocations by service								

212 / Appendix A

HOSPITAL GOVERNANCE

The following questions concern your hospital's governing board.

11. Name the bodies (Regents, Hospital Trustees, Adivsory Boards/Committees) your have that are involved in governance decisions.

    ☐ _____
    ☐ _____
    ☐ _____
    ☐ _____

12. Which of the above comes closest to <u>functioning</u> as the true operational board of your hospital? Please indicate by placing a check ☑ next to it.

EXTREMELY IMPORTANT ⟶ *IN THE QUESTIONS TO FOLLOW, ASSUME THE WORD "BOARD" REFERS TO THE BODY YOU CHECKED ☑ ABOVE AS BEING THE HOSPITAL'S OPERATIONAL BOARD. ⟵ EXTREMELY IMPORTANT

13. How many voting members does this Board* have? _____

14. How are members of your Board* selected?

    _____ Elected (specify how many) _____
    _____ Appointed (specify how many and who appoints) _____
    _____ Ex-officio, i.e., serve on Board* <u>with</u> <u>vote</u> because they hold some other office (specify how many) _____

15. How many "outsiders" are on your Board*, i.e., those who are <u>not</u> employees or officials of the state or any of its agencies, the university or any of its divisions. _____

16. What is the occupation and title (if retired, give last position held) of the person now serving as Chairman of your Board*? _____

17. How is the Chairman selected and/or appointed?

    _____ Elected by members of the Board*
    _____ Appointed by _____
    _____ Bylaws specify the Board* member holding the following position shall also serve as Chairman of the Board* _____
    _____ Other (specify) _____

18. How many years has this Board been in operation? _____ (years)

19. In which area is the Board* most effective (check only one):

    _____ The Board's* contribution is in providing a linkage (and buffer) to demands of the state or the university administration or the medical school or others who have a sense of ownership of the hospital. <u>It protects our ability to manage.</u>
    _____ The Board's* contribution is in helping negotiations with or influence regulatory groups, or reimbursers, or capital or gift sources, or the public. <u>It helps us get resources.</u>
    _____ The Board's* contribution is in setting direction (e.g., long range planning), and keeping track of progress. <u>It helps us stay on course.</u>
    _____ The Board's* contribution is in performing certain legal functions (e.g., quality monitoring, medical staff appointment approval) and assisting in other ways. <u>It helps in the effective management of the hospital.</u>

20. Which statements describe <u>best</u> and <u>second best</u> how the Board* operates? (Put 1 against the "best" statement, and 2 against the "second best" statement.)

   _____ Initiates plans and proposals, and influences the process by which decisions about them are made.
   _____ Works collaboratively with university and hospital official(s) in developing plans and proposals and controlling the decision process.
   _____ Creatively reacts to proposals of university and hospital official(s).
   _____ Typically endorses proposals referred to them.

21. Which statements describe <u>best</u> and <u>second best</u> the content of Board* discussions and decisions? (Rank in manner as above.)

   _____ Strategic, long-range, policy-type matters, i.e., "governance" matters.
   _____ Operational, shorter-range, more procedural matters, i.e., "management."
   _____ Deals with approximately equal proportions of governance and management.

22. How effective is your Board*?

   _____ Highly effective
   _____ Effective
   _____ Mixed, varies by the issue over time
   _____ Ineffective

23. List three major actions taken by your Board* and the years they were taken:

   1. _____ Year _____

   2. _____ Year _____

   3. _____ Year _____

24. On balance, when Board* members are making decisions, whose interests are they thinking of? To whom do they owe their loyalty?

   _____ Thinking primarily of satisfying the officer that selected them.
   _____ Thinking primarily of representing the interests of the unit or organization they manage or work in, and which qualified them to serve on this Board*.
   _____ Thinking primarily of representing the interests of the medical center as a whole.
   _____ Thinking primarily of representing the interests of the hospital as a whole.
   _____ None of the above.

Background and Environmental Information

25. What approximate percent of your patients come from the following areas:

   (a) your immediate community ____%; (b) surrounding communities ____%; (c) outside these areas ____%.

IMPORTANT ➤ For the questions to follow assume your answers to questions 25 (a) and (b) identify your primary service area.

26. What is the percent of the population change in your primary service area over the past five years?

   Down ⟩ _____ less than 5%   Up ⟩ _____ less than 5%   _____ No Change
         _____ more than 5%   _____ more than 5%

27. a) How many hospitals are there in this primary service area? _____
    b) How many of these hospitals would you consider to be competitive with yours? _____

28. Are the following facilities available in your primary service area (<u>excluding</u> your own hospital)?

   YES   NO
   ___   ___   Teaching hospitals
   ___   ___   Tertiary care medical centers
   ___   ___   County hospitals
   ___   ___   Multi-hospital systems
   ___   ___   Major private practice medical groups that include specialists who depend on referral practice
   ___   ___   Large HMO practice
   ___   ___   Large IPAs

29. How would you describe changes in the economic conditions of your state in the last five years?

    _____ Has gotten significantly worse
    _____ Has gotten worse
    _____ Has stayed about the same
    _____ Has gotten better
    _____ Has gotten significantly better

30. How predictable, compared to two to three years ago, are the actions of regulators in:

	More Predictable	No Change	Less Predictable
capital expansion	_____	_____	_____
capital replacement	_____	_____	_____
corporate restructuring	_____	_____	_____
Blue Cross reimbursement	_____	_____	_____
Medicaid	_____	_____	_____
Other government reimbursement	_____	_____	_____

31. Relative to other competitive hospitals in your area, how supportive are the regulators of your hospital?

    _____ Not appropriate, no other competing hospital around
    _____ More supportive of our hospital than others
    _____ Less supportive of our hospital than others
    _____ About the same

32. On balance, the number of groups or agencies whose cooperation is needed before regulatory approval is obtained for similar CON applications are:

    _____ More numerous than two years ago
    _____ Less numerous than two years ago
    _____ About the same as two years ago

33. On balance, the complexity of procedures involved with outside groups to obtain support/approval:

    _____ Is simpler than two years ago
    _____ Is more complex than two years ago
    _____ Is about the same

34. To what extent have hospitals in your service area changed the nature of their corporate structure in the last five years?

	Trend toward	No change	Trend away from
multi-institutional affiliation	_____	_____	_____
mergers	_____	_____	_____
contract management services	_____	_____	_____
joint ventures	_____	_____	_____
HMO contract sources	_____	_____	_____

35. Rate the amount of high-level administrative attention required in dealing with the following agencies or groups:

	Insignificant High-level Attention	Occasional High-level Attention	Considerable High-level Attention	Very Much High-level Attention
Reimbursers:				
BC/BS	_____	_____	_____	_____
Medicare	_____	_____	_____	_____
Medicaid	_____	_____	_____	_____
Commercial Insurers	_____	_____	_____	_____
Regulatory/Review:				
HSAs	_____	_____	_____	_____
Rate Review	_____	_____	_____	_____
Licensing Authorities	_____	_____	_____	_____
JCAH	_____	_____	_____	_____
Safety/Sanitation Inspectors	_____	_____	_____	_____
Other Health Care Organizations:				
HMOs	_____	_____	_____	_____
Local Hospital Council	_____	_____	_____	_____
State/National Associations	_____	_____	_____	_____

36. What percent of your patient charges are:

   Unreimbursed, or written off _____%;
   Covered by state appropriations _____%

37. How strong is the state expectation that your hospital will care for government-sponsored patients other than Medicare?

   _____ Mandatory
   _____ Virtually mandatory
   _____ Expected
   _____ Optional

38. What is the image of your hospital in the community?

	Not seen this way	Somewhat seen this way	Strongly seen this way
A place for indigent care	_____	_____	_____
A place for community care	_____	_____	_____
A place for highly specialized care	_____	_____	_____

39. What proportion of your active physicians have affiliations with other hospitals?

   _____ 0%
   _____ 1-25%
   _____ 26-50%
   _____ 51-75%
   _____ 76+%

40. Give us your best estimate of the immediate future of your hospital.

	Quite Likely	Possibly	Unlikely	No	Not Applicable
A. Will you attract all the ambulatory patients you want?	_____	_____	_____	_____	_____
B. Will you attract all the normal care inpatients you want?	_____	_____	_____	_____	_____
C. Will you attract all the tertiary care patients you want?	_____	_____	_____	_____	_____
D. Will rate review show a reasonable recognition of the special needs of university hospital operations?	_____	_____	_____	_____	_____
E. Will Blue Cross show a reasonable recognition of the special needs of university hospital operations?	_____	_____	_____	_____	_____
F. Will Medicaid show a reasonable recognition of the special needs of university hospital operations?	_____	_____	_____	_____	_____
G. Will Medicare show a reasonable recognition of the special needs of university hospital operations?	_____	_____	_____	_____	_____
H. Will health planning agencies show a reasonable recognition of the special needs of university hospital operations?	_____	_____	_____	_____	_____
I. Will other major hospitals cooperate with you in rationally meeting the care needs of your service area?	_____	_____	_____	_____	_____
J. Will other hospitals aggressively seek to capture major components of your current patient population?	_____	_____	_____	_____	_____
K. Will reduction in education or research funding result in the hospital bearing more of these costs?	_____	_____	_____	_____	_____
L. Will the university actively support needed hospital expansion?	_____	_____	_____	_____	_____
M. Will the state supply capital for needed hospital expansion?	_____	_____	_____	_____	_____
N. Will the state cooperate in arranging lower interest rates on hospital borrowing?	_____	_____	_____	_____	_____
O. Will the community support a capital gifts campaign?	_____	_____	_____	_____	_____

Exact name of your hospital _____

"COTH publishes financial and operating data from your hospital and other member hospitals. Rather than collect this same information from you for our survey, we are asking for your permission to use the COTH data. COTH has generously agreed to let us use these data with your permission. Please indicate your approval by signing on the line below."

Date _____ Signature _____

Thank you very much for completing this questionnaire. Your help is very much appreciated. If you have additional comments of any nature you wish to convey to us, please write in below.

APPENDIX B

Survey and Field Study Respondents

HOSPITALS THAT COMPLETED THE CSUH SURVEY

University of Alabama Hospitals
Birmingham, AL

University of South Alabama
Medical Center Hospital
Mobile, AL

University Hospital
University of Arizona
Tucson, AZ

University Hospital
University of Arkansas
Little Rock, AR

Loma Linda University Medical
Center
Loma Linda, CA

*U.C.L.A. Hospital and Clinics
Los Angeles, CA

University of California, Davis
Sacramento Medical Center
Sacramento, CA

*University of California
Hospitals, San Francisco
San Francisco, CA

Field study hospitals are shown with *. Johns Hopkins Hospital, Baltimore, MD, was a field study hospital in addition to those marked with an * above. It is not a university-owned hospital and was not surveyed.

Stanford University Medical Center
Stanford, CA

*University Hospital
University of Colorado
Denver, CO

University of Connecticut Health Center
John Dempsey Hospital
Farmington, CT

George Washington University Hospital
Washington, DC

Georgetown University Hospital
Washington, DC

*William A. Shands Teaching Hospital
University of Florida
Gainesville, FL

Crawford W. Long Memorial Hospital
Emory University
Atlanta, GA

Emory University Hospital
Atlanta, GA

Eugene Talmadge Memorial Hospital
Medical College of Georgia
Augusta, GA

University of Chicago
Hospitals and Clinics
Chicago, IL

University of Illinois Hospital
Chicago, IL

Foster G. McGaw Hospital
Loyola University
Maywood, IL

Indiana University Hospitals
Indianapolis, IN

*University of Iowa
Hospitals and Clinics
Iowa City, IA

University of Kansas
Medical Center
Kansas City, KS

*Albert B. Chandler Medical Center
University of Kentucky
Lexington, KY

Confederate Memorial Medical Center
Louisiana State University
Shreveport, LA

University of Maryland Hospital
Baltimore, MD

*University of Massachusetts Hospital
Worcester, MA

*University Hospital
University of Michigan
Ann Arbor, MI

*University of Minnesota
Hospitals and Clinics
Minneapolis, MN

University Hospital
University of Mississippi
Jackson, MS

University of Missouri
Medical Center
Columbia, MO

St. Louis University Hospitals
St. Louis, MO

*University of Nebraska
Medical Center
Omaha, NE

UMDNJ College Hospital
Newark, NJ

New York University
Medical Center
New York, NY

*Strong Memorial Hospital
of the University of Rochester
Rochester, NY

*North Carolina Memorial Hospital
Chapel Hill, NC

Cincinnati General Hospital
University of Cincinnati
Cincinnati, OH

University Hospital
University of Oregon
Health Sciences Center
Portland, OR

The Milton S. Hershey Medical
Center
Pennsylvania State University
Hershey, PA

Hahnemann Medical College
and Hospital of Philadelphia
Philadelphia, PA

Medical College of Pennsylvania
and Hospital
Philadelphia, PA

Thomas Jefferson University
Hospital
Philadelphia, PA

Temple University Hospital
Philadelphia, PA

Medical University Hospital
Medical University of South Carolina
Charleston, SC

Vanderbilt University Hospital
Nashville, TN

University of Virginia Hospitals
Charlottesville, VA

*Medical College of Virginia
Hospitals
Richmond, VA

*University of Washington Hospitals
Seattle, WA

West Virginia University Hospital
Morgantown, WV

University of Wisconsin Hospitals
Madison, WI

Index

Academic health centers (AHCs): administration, 188; AHC board or hospital board, 181; AHC/hospital board as a management and governance mode, 177–78
Adaptability, 203
Administration. *See* Hospital administration
Admissions, 7, 125, 132
Appropriation-independent hospitals, 194
Appropriations, 30, 118, 128, 182, 183, 184, 193, 194, 195, 204–5; and board age, 46; and board effectiveness, 48–49; and board function, 46–47; and board proactivity, 47; and centralization of governance decision making, 48; and dispersion of power in governance decision making, 47–48; and governance structure, 45–46; and management variables, 176; and relationship between political culture and hospital dependence on appropriations, 78
Aston studies, 79–80
Autonomy: of hospitals, 180, 181, 198; of universities, 72

Bed: inventory per occupied, 139; personnel per, 139
Blue Cross, 118
Business climate, 75; index, 68–69

Capital: financing, 7; funds, 81; structure, 120, 122, 123
Case mix, 7, 125–26; and costs, 118
Centralization, 186, 192
CEO, 196; managerial influence, 92, 93; tenure, 6, 86, 87; tenure affected by state environment, 86, 92, 93; turnover, 92, 93
Charity, 6, 11, 78, 79, 81. *See also* Indigent care; Welfare

222 / Index

Clinical chiefs, 200–201
Clinical faculty reimbursement, 157, 158, 159
Collection rates, 7
Commercialization of university hospitals, 3, 196
Competition, 2, 7, 8, 68, 102, 111, 156, 169, 184, 185, 186; affected by appropriations, 112; and control, 153; and cost control, 9–15; and efficiency, 103; and indigent care, 104; local, 86, 87, 110; and regulation in "moralistic" states, 81; state (impact on viability), 89, 90; state and local, 107; and viability, 103. *See also* Environment: competitive
Consortium for the Study of University Hospitals (CSUH): formation, xiii; Survey of the Management and Governance of University-Owned Teaching Hospitals, Appendix A, 207–16
Costs, 127–28
CSUH Survey participants, Appendix B, 217–19

Data analysis, 102; correlations, scaling/indexing, path analysis, 20–23; of financial viability, 123, 124, 125, 126, 127, 128, 129, 130, 131, 132, 133; of impact of environment on university hospital performance, 105–7; limitations, 23–25
Data sources, 4, 19–20, 72–73; for support services, 138
Debt financing, 118
Decentralization, 194–95
DRGs, 113, 164, 187, 195, 196, 197; and indigent care, 92. *See also* Prospective payment

Education level, 127
Efficiency, 5, 6, 7, 17, 104, 127, 169, 181, 182; associated with state influence, 79; in resource utilization, 139; and viability related to environmental and organizational variables, 99, 100, 101, 102
Environment, 13, 191; competitive, 12, 18–19; competitive vs. protective, 18; impact on university hospital performance, 105–7; internal, 5, 12; market, 5, 28, 191; market and political and governance structure, 41–42; ownership, 5, 8, 12, 18–19, 184, 191, 205; political, 5, 12, 28, 192; political and its effect on hospital governance, 67; state, 114; state (affecting hospital viability), 88, 89, 90, 93, 94; state (as a combination of competitive and political environment), 85; state (with local competition as a variable), 86; state (stratified by proactivism, state competition, and local competition), 87–88; task, 12

Federal subsidies, 203
Financial management decisions, 198

Governing boards, 8, 114, 163–64, 174, 199, 200, 201, 202, 203; effectiveness, 40–41; emphasis on governance or management, 35–36; external/internal orientation, 34–35, 177, 181; orientation compared with environment, 42; proactivism, 36–37, 41–42, 102; size, 33–34; type, 32–33
Gross patient revenues, 127, 129
Group practice, 157

HMOs, 10, 187
Hospital administration, 175–76; and board power, 177, 181; externally oriented, 102, 111, 177, 181;

externally oriented and hospital performance, 103; externally oriented and proactive governance, 102–3; via a strong board, 189; in a strong role, 188–89

Hospital performance, 6–7, 54; definition of, 54; efficiency and viability as criteria, 54–55; internal process perspective, 57; judging effectiveness via four perspectives, 55–56; measurement data, 58; measuring, 5–6, 13; measuring resource efficiency, 59; organizational goals perspective, 56; related to political culture, 78; strategic constituencies perspective, 58; system-resource perspective, 56–57; weakness in data, 59

Hospital performance variables: efficiency, 61; facilities, 62; patients per house officer, 62; relationships among performance indexes, 62–65; viability, 59–61

Hospital size, 7, 30, 31, 120, 122, 127, 133; related to governance structure, 45

Indigent care, 7, 86, 87, 91, 92, 107, 108, 109, 110, 126, 129, 134, 154, 155, 156, 160, 193; affected by state environment, 86; and competition, 104; and hospital efficiency and viability, 104; and medical school ranking, 104; and performance, 104–5. *See also* Charity; Welfare

Innovations, 204

Interdependence among hospital and other university units, 143

Inventory per occupied bed, 139

Key group decision making, 37–40; influence of, 177, 178, 179, 180

Leadership, 194; strong vs. weak, 183–84

Linkage of hospitals, 96

"Loose coupling," 18

Management, participative, 167

Management process: clarity in decision making, 167–69, 170; "dominant personality" and "political" approaches, 168, 169; executive and collegial approaches, 168, 169

Managerial competence, 143–44

Managerial decisions, 127, 132

Managerial and governance characteristics compared, 197

Managerial and governance conflicts, 8

Medicaid, 118, 134

Medical school administration vs. clinical chiefs, 175

Medical school prestige, 107

Medical school ranking, 114; and hospital performance, 104; and indigent care, 104

Medical service plans (MSPs), 157, 158, 159, 160

Medical staff characteristics, 125

Medical staff governance, 161; "bicameral" mode, 161–62; chief of staff, 162–63; "strong dean," 161–62; vice-president for health services ("corporate" model), 163

Medical staff organization, 8, 151

Medicare, 118, 134

Multihospital chains, 2, 3, 10

Multiunit systems, 203–4

Occupancy, 120, 123; growth-adjusted, 139

Open systems theory, 12

Ownership, 125, 191, 192, 193; of hospitals, 1, 30, 31; and managerial influence, 133; and viability, 133

Ownership—public or private: advantages and disadvantages, 81–82; and board function, 43; and "centralized" and "decentralized" hospitals, 43–44; correlated with governance structure measures, 42–43; and dispersion of influence in governance, 44–45; as an environmental factor, 80; related to political subculture, 76–78; related to population-ecology and protected-organization perspectives, 80

Patient care, 8, 151–53, 169, 200; control structures, 166–67; decisions influenced by different officials, 165–66; policy decisions, 198–99
Payment source, 7, 127
Performance, 193
Personnel per bed, 139
Policy implications: of contextual variables, 50–51; of ownership and appropriations, 50–51
"Political culture," 69–71, 73, 74, 75, 76; related to governance, 78–79; subcultures—"moralist" ("commonwealth"), "elitist" ("traditionalist"), and "individualist" ("market"), 70–71; subcultures related to environment variables, 73
Politically progressive states compared with conservative states, 193
Population-ecology model, 16
Privately and publicly owned university hospitals compared, 7
Proactive/competitive states (ranking), 29
Proactive states: appropriations, 103; indigent care, 91–92; medical school ranking, 103; university independence, 102
Proactivity, 3, 5, 28

Profitability, 120, 122–23
Prospective payment, 8, 10. *See also* DRGs
Protected-organizations perspective, 17

Research, 119, 152, 155, 160, 193, 200, 201
Residency training, 11
Resource-dependence perspective, 14
Revenue deduction rate, 127
Revenues, 7; gross patient, 127, 129; and receivables, 139
Revenue source, 30, 79

Shared service systems, 10
Specialty referral center (SRC), 118–19
State influence on university hospitals, 173
Subsidies, federal, 203
Support services, 7, 137, 139, 140, 141, 142, 145–47, 149–50; academic health center control, 141; association between hospital control and performance, 139–42; control at higher levels, 142; degree of hospital control, 140; distribution of control, 141; Kerr's strategy for securing, 147–49; monitored and provided by university units, 144; multiple control and hospital efficiency, 141–42
Systematic relationships: correlation of four contextual variables with seven governance variables, 27–29

Teaching, 6–7, 10, 119, 200, 201; effect on viability and efficiency, 111–12; related to costs and utilization, 118

Teaching hospital: primary, 10
Tertiary care, 3, 78, 113, 129, 134, 195, 204

University administration of hospitals, 188
University hospital organization, 11
University hospitals: as commercial for-profit organization, 113–14; operating in an enterprise mode, 146–47; organization, 11; as separate corporations, 96, 114, 146; structure: functional or product-type, 164–65
University independence and proactive governance, 102
University influence on their hospitals, 174

Viability, 5–6, 7, 14–15, 17, 20, 107; affected by state environment, 86; affected by state proactivism and competition, 88, 89, 90; enhancement of, 94, 95, 96; financial, 118, 120, 123–25

Wages, 125
Welfare, 7, 72, 73–75; and hospital viability and efficiency, 104; paid by state, 181; and proactive states, 103. *See also* Charity; Indigent care

About the Authors

THOMAS CHOI, PH.D., is associate professor and head, Section of Hospitals and Interorganizational Studies at the Center for Health Services Research, School of Public Health, University of Minnesota. He holds additional appointments in the Graduate Program in Hospital and Health Care Administration, Social and Administrative Pharmacy, and the Department of Sociology. Professor Choi has published articles regarding university hospitals in *Medical Care* and *Health Care Management Review*. He teaches graduate courses in advanced measurement techniques in social research and organizational theory as applied to the health care setting.

ROBERT ALLISON, PH.D., Associate Professor of Management at Wayne State University, has taught, done research, and published in health services administration. He also has had experience as a health care executive ranging from small community hospitals to The University of Michigan Hospitals where he served as Associate to the Director. Noteworthy among his research contributions are his work on the roles of administrators in hospitals, clinics, nursing homes, and HMOs, as well as his investigations in one of seven studies on prospective reimbursement funded by the Social Security Administration. Dr. Allison is a member of the American College of Healthcare Executives and is active in the Academy of Management.

FRED MUNSON, PH.D., is a professor of Hospital Administration at The University of Michigan's School of Public Health, where he teaches organization theory and the design of health care organizations. In recent years his research has been on the management and governance of academic health centers and the design and/or restructuring of multihospital systems. Prior to that his research addressed issues more internal to hospital organizations, such as unit management and nursing unit organization design, and problems of implementing innovations. He remains active in two other fields of long-standing interest: labor-management relations, where he continues to act as an impartial arbitrator, and Indian health care, where he, along with his wife, assists nonprofit hospitals by training, consultation, or other means.

DATE DUE

GAYLORD　　　　　　　　　　　　　　PRINTED IN U.S.A.